NO GALLBLADE COOKBOOK

The Ultimate Guide to Transform Your Eating Experience After Removal. Nourish Your Body with Easy and Simple Recipes and a 28-Day Meal Plan for Optimal Digestive Health.

+2 Bonus inside the book

+ Color Version of the book

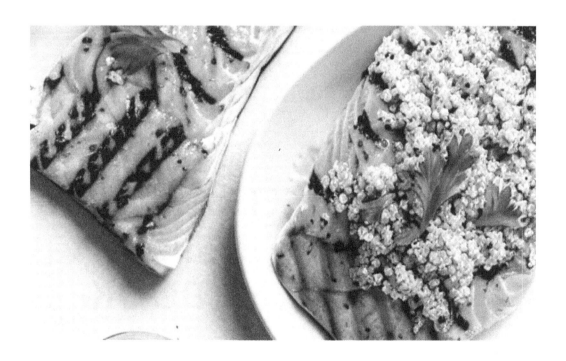

William C. Dean

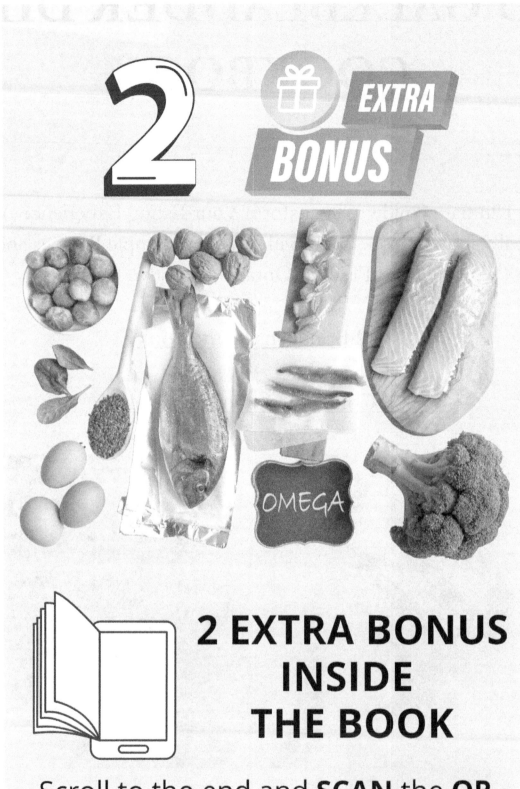

2 EXTRA BONUS
INSIDE
THE BOOK

Scroll to the end and **SCAN** the **QR CODE** to dowload the **2 FREE BONUS**

Table of Contents

Introduction

The No Gallbladder Diet Cookbook is designed to help individuals who have had their gallbladder removed navigate the dietary changes they need to make in order to maintain a healthy and balanced diet. The absence of a gallbladder can cause digestive problems, and it is important to make certain dietary adjustments in order to minimize symptoms and prevent further complications.

This cookbook provides a comprehensive guide to the no gallbladder diet, including an overview of the benefits of following this type of diet, as well as tips for selecting and storing ingredients. The recipes in this cookbook are designed to be easy to prepare, delicious, and suitable for those following a no gallbladder diet. From breakfast dishes to snacks and desserts, this cookbook has something for everyone.

Whether you are new to the no gallbladder diet or have been following it for some time, this cookbook is an essential resource for maintaining a healthy and balanced diet. With its wide variety of recipes and helpful tips, it provides everything you need to stay on track and feel your best.

Explanation of the purpose of the book

The purpose of the No Gallbladder Diet Cookbook is to provide individuals who have had their gallbladder removed with the tools and information they need to maintain a healthy and balanced diet. The absence of a gallbladder can impact the digestive process, and it is important to make certain dietary adjustments in order to minimize symptoms and prevent further complications.

This cookbook is designed to make it easy for individuals to follow a no gallbladder diet by providing a wide variety of delicious, easy-to-prepare recipes. The recipes in this cookbook have been created with the unique needs of those without a gallbladder in mind, and are carefully balanced to ensure that they provide all the nutrients needed for optimal health.

In addition to the recipes, this cookbook includes important information about the no gallbladder diet, including an overview of the digestive process without a gallbladder and the recommended dietary changes for people without a gallbladder. With its comprehensive approach, the No Gallbladder Diet Cookbook is the ultimate resource for anyone looking to maintain a healthy diet after having their gallbladder removed.

Overview of the no gallbladder diet

The no gallbladder diet is a type of diet specifically designed for individuals who have had their gallbladder removed. The gallbladder is an important organ that helps the body store and release bile, which is a digestive juice that helps break down fats. When the gallbladder is removed, the body must find a new way to process fats, which can result in digestive problems.

The no gallbladder diet is designed to minimize these problems by limiting the amount of fat in the diet and recommending certain foods and preparation methods that are easier on the digestive system. This type of diet typically includes a variety of lean proteins, whole grains, fruits, and vegetables, as well as low-fat dairy products and healthy fats like olive oil.

In addition to the recommended foods, the no gallbladder diet also includes guidelines for portion sizes and meal frequency, as well as tips for avoiding common trigger foods that can cause digestive problems. It is important to note that the no gallbladder diet may vary from person to person, and it is recommended to work with a healthcare provider or registered dietitian to create a personalized plan that meets your specific needs and goals.

By following a no gallbladder diet, individuals can help minimize symptoms and prevent further complications, as well as maintain a healthy and balanced diet. This cookbook provides a comprehensive guide to the no gallbladder diet, including a variety of delicious and easy-to-prepare recipes, making it the ultimate resource for anyone looking to maintain a healthy diet after having their gallbladder removed.

Benefits of following a no gallbladder diet

Following a no gallbladder diet offers numerous benefits for individuals who have had their gallbladder removed. Some of the key benefits include:

Minimizing digestive problems: One of the main benefits of the no gallbladder diet is that it can help minimize digestive problems caused by the absence of a gallbladder. By limiting the amount of fat in the diet and including certain foods that are easier on the digestive system, individuals can help reduce symptoms like bloating, gas, and diarrhea.

Promoting overall health: The no gallbladder diet is designed to include a variety of nutrient-rich foods that are essential for optimal health, such as lean proteins, whole grains, fruits, and vegetables, as well as low-fat dairy products and healthy fats. By following this type of diet, individuals can help ensure they are getting all the nutrients they need for overall health and well-being.

Improving cholesterol levels: The no gallbladder diet typically includes foods that are low in unhealthy fats and high in healthy fats, which can help improve cholesterol levels and reduce the risk of heart disease.

Supporting weight management: The no gallbladder diet is designed to be balanced and nutrient-rich, which can help support weight management. By limiting portion sizes and including a variety of healthy foods, individuals can help maintain a healthy weight and prevent weight gain.

Improving energy levels: The no gallbladder diet includes foods that provide sustained energy, such as whole grains, fruits, and vegetables, which can help improve energy levels throughout the day.

By following a no gallbladder diet, individuals can enjoy numerous benefits for their health and well-being. With its comprehensive approach, the No Gallbladder Diet Cookbook provides everything you need to maintain a healthy and balanced diet after having your gallbladder removed.

Explanation of the cookbook format and structure

The No Gallbladder Diet Cookbook is designed to be a comprehensive and user-friendly resource for individuals who have had their gallbladder removed. The cookbook is structured as follows:

Introduction: This section provides an overview of the purpose of the book, including important information about the no gallbladder diet and its benefits.

Overview of the No Gallbladder Diet: This chapter provides a detailed explanation of the no gallbladder diet, including the recommended foods, portion sizes, meal frequency, and tips for avoiding trigger foods.

Recipes: The core of the cookbook, this section includes a wide variety of delicious and easy-to-prepare recipes that have been specifically designed for individuals following a no gallbladder diet. The recipes are organized by meal type, including breakfast, lunch, dinner, snacks, and desserts, making it easy to find the perfect recipe for any occasion.

Nutritional Information: Each recipe in the cookbook includes a comprehensive nutritional analysis, including information on calories, fat, protein, fiber, and other key nutrients, making it easy to track your dietary intake.

Conclusion: The final section of the cookbook includes additional tips and resources for maintaining a healthy no gallbladder diet, as well as suggestions for further reading and research.

The No Gallbladder Diet Cookbook is designed to be an all-in-one resource for individuals looking to maintain a healthy and balanced diet after having their gallbladder removed. With its comprehensive approach and delicious recipes, this cookbook is the ultimate tool for anyone looking to improve their health and well-being.

Understanding the No Gallbladder Diet

The no gallbladder diet is a type of diet that is recommended for individuals who have had their gallbladder removed. The primary goal of this diet is to help minimize digestive problems and promote overall health and well-being.

The gallbladder is a small, pear-shaped organ that is responsible for storing and releasing bile, which is a digestive enzyme that helps break down fats in the small intestine. Without a gallbladder, the liver releases bile directly into the small intestine, which can sometimes result in digestive problems.

To help minimize these issues, the no gallbladder diet is designed to limit the amount of fat in the diet and to include certain foods that are easier on the digestive system. The diet typically includes lean proteins, whole grains, fruits, vegetables, low-fat dairy products, and healthy fats, while avoiding high-fat and high-cholesterol foods.

It is also important for individuals following a no gallbladder diet to limit their portion sizes, eat frequent small meals throughout the day, and to avoid or limit trigger foods that can cause digestive problems. Trigger foods can vary from person to person, but may include fatty or greasy foods, fried foods, spicy foods, and carbonated drinks.

By following the no gallbladder diet, individuals can help minimize digestive problems and promote overall health and well-being. The No Gallbladder Diet Cookbook provides all the information and tools you need to successfully follow this type of diet and enjoy a variety of delicious and nutritious meals.

Definition of a gallbladder

The gallbladder is a small, pear-shaped organ located on the right side of the abdomen, just below the liver. Its primary function is to store and release bile, a digestive enzyme that helps to break down fats in the small intestine. Bile is produced by the liver and is stored in the gallbladder until it is needed for digestion.

The gallbladder works in coordination with the liver and the small intestine to help digest and absorb fats and other nutrients. When food enters the small intestine, signals are sent to the gallbladder to release bile into the small intestine. The bile then emulsifies the fat, breaking it down into smaller particles that can be more easily absorbed by the body.

In some cases, individuals may have their gallbladder removed due to medical conditions such as gallstones, inflammation of the gallbladder, or other complications. After the gallbladder is removed, the liver still produces bile, but it is released directly into the small intestine rather than being stored in the gallbladder.

It is important for individuals who have had their gallbladder removed to follow a special diet, known as the no gallbladder diet, in order to minimize digestive problems and promote overall health and well being. The No Gallbladder Diet Cookbook provides all the information and tools you need to successfully follow this type of diet and enjoy a variety of delicious and nutritious meals.

Explanation of why the gallbladder is removed

The gallbladder is removed for a variety of medical reasons, including:

Gallstones: Gallstones are hard deposits of bile that can form in the gallbladder. These stones can cause pain and discomfort, as well as block the bile ducts and cause other complications. In cases of severe or recurrent gallstones, removal of the gallbladder may be recommended.

Inflammation of the Gallbladder: Inflammation of the gallbladder, also known as cholecystitis, can be caused by a variety of factors, including infection, obstruction of the bile ducts, or other medical conditions. In some cases, chronic inflammation of the gallbladder may lead to removal of the organ.

Other Complications: Other medical conditions, such as cancer of the gallbladder or bile ducts, can also lead to removal of the gallbladder. In these cases, removal of the gallbladder may be necessary to prevent the spread of disease or to preserve overall health and well-being.

Regardless of the reason for removal, it is important for individuals who have had their gallbladder removed to follow a special diet, known as the no gallbladder diet, in order to minimize digestive problems and promote overall health and well-being. The No Gallbladder Diet Cookbook provides all the information and tools you need to successfully follow this type of diet and enjoy a variety of delicious and nutritious meals.

Overview of the digestive process without a gallbladder

The digestive process without a gallbladder differs slightly from the digestive process with a functioning gallbladder. In individuals with a functioning gallbladder, bile is stored in the organ and is released as needed to help digest and absorb fats and other nutrients.

However, in individuals who have had their gallbladder removed, the liver still produces bile, but it is released directly into the small intestine rather than being stored in the gallbladder. This change in the digestive process can sometimes result in digestive problems, including diarrhea, abdominal pain, and bloating.

To help minimize these issues, individuals who have had their gallbladder removed are often advised to follow a special diet, known as the no gallbladder diet. This type of diet is designed to limit the amount of fat in the diet and to include certain foods that are easier on the digestive system.

It is also important for individuals following a no gallbladder diet to limit their portion sizes, eat frequent small meals throughout the day, and to avoid or limit trigger foods that can cause digestive problems. By following these guidelines, individuals can help minimize digestive problems and promote overall health and well-being.

The No Gallbladder Diet Cookbook provides all the information and tools you need to successfully follow the no gallbladder diet and enjoy a variety of delicious and nutritious meals.

Explanation of the recommended dietary changes for people without a gallbladder

Individuals who have had their gallbladder removed are often advised to make certain dietary changes in order to minimize digestive problems and promote overall health and well-being. Some of the recommended changes include:

Limit Fat: A key aspect of the no gallbladder diet is to limit the amount of fat in the diet. This is because without the gallbladder to store and release bile, the body may have a harder time digesting fats. It is recommended to limit fat intake to 20-30 grams per meal.

Increase Fiber: Increasing fiber in the diet can help regulate digestion and prevent constipation, a common problem for individuals without a gallbladder. It is recommended to eat plenty of fruits, vegetables, whole grains, and legumes.

Avoid Trigger Foods: Certain foods, such as fatty foods, spicy foods, and carbonated drinks, can trigger digestive problems in individuals without a gallbladder. It is important to avoid or limit these trigger foods in order to minimize digestive issues.

Eat Small, Frequent Meals: Eating small, frequent meals throughout the day can help regulate digestion and prevent symptoms such as abdominal pain and bloating. It is recommended to eat 5-6 small meals per day rather than 3 large meals.

Drink Plenty of Water: Drinking plenty of water is important for overall health and can also help regulate digestion in individuals without a gallbladder. It is recommended to drink at least 8 glasses of water per day.

By following these dietary recommendations, individuals without a gallbladder can minimize digestive problems and promote overall health and well-being. The No Gallbladder Diet Cookbook provides a variety of delicious and nutritious meal options that are specifically designed for individuals following the no gallbladder diet.

Ingredients and Equipment

List of recommended ingredients for a no gallbladder diet

When following a no gallbladder diet, it is important to include a variety of nutritious and easy-to-digest foods in your meals. Some of the recommended ingredients for this type of diet include:

Lean protein: sources of lean protein include chicken, fish, tofu, and legumes.

Fruits and vegetables: fiber-rich fruits and vegetables, such as apples, berries, leafy greens, and carrots, can help regulate digestion and prevent constipation.

Whole grains: choose whole grain breads, pastas, and cereals for added fiber and nutrition.

Low-fat dairy: low-fat dairy products, such as milk, yogurt, and cheese, can provide calcium and other important nutrients.

Healthy fats: sources of healthy fats include avocado, nuts, and olive oil.

Herbs and spices: herbs and spices, such as ginger and turmeric, can help regulate digestion and add flavor to meals.

By incorporating these recommended ingredients into your meals, you can create delicious and nutritious meals that support your health and well-being. The No Gallbladder Diet Cookbook includes a variety of recipes that incorporate these recommended ingredients to make following the no gallbladder diet easy and enjoyable.

Explanation of the use of each ingredient

Lean protein: Lean protein is important for overall health and provides the body with essential nutrients. The body requires protein to build and repair tissues, maintain a healthy immune system, and regulate metabolism. In a no gallbladder diet, it is important to choose lean protein sources, as high-fat protein sources can be difficult for the body to digest without a gallbladder.

Fruits and vegetables: Fruits and vegetables are rich in fiber, vitamins, and minerals. Fiber helps regulate digestion and prevent constipation, while vitamins and minerals support overall health and well-being. Eating a variety of colorful fruits and vegetables can also add flavor and nutrition to meals.

Whole grains: Whole grains are a good source of fiber, vitamins, and minerals. They can help regulate digestion and prevent constipation, and they also provide energy and keep you feeling full. Whole grains are a healthier option compared to refined grains, which have had the fiber removed.

Low-fat dairy: Low-fat dairy products provide calcium and other important nutrients, such as vitamin D and protein. Calcium is important for strong bones, and vitamin D helps the body absorb calcium. In a no gallbladder diet, it is recommended to choose low-fat dairy products, as high-fat dairy products can be difficult for the body to digest.

Healthy fats: Healthy fats, such as avocado, nuts, and olive oil, are important for overall health and provide the body with energy. They also help regulate digestion and keep you feeling full. In a no gallbladder diet, it is recommended to limit fat intake, but including a small amount of healthy fats in your diet can be beneficial.

Herbs and spices: Herbs and spices not only add flavor to meals, but they also have a variety of health benefits. For example, ginger has been shown to help regulate digestion, while turmeric has anti-inflammatory properties. Incorporating a variety of herbs and spices into your meals can add flavor and support your health.

By incorporating these recommended ingredients into your meals, you can create delicious and nutritious meals that support your health and well-being. The No Gallbladder Diet Cookbook provides a variety of recipes that incorporate these recommended ingredients to make following the no gallbladder diet easy and enjoyable.

Essential kitchen equipment for preparing no gallbladder diet meals

Having the right kitchen equipment is essential for preparing nutritious and delicious meals that support a no gallbladder diet. Some of the essential kitchen equipment for preparing no gallbladder diet meals include:

Cutting boards: a set of cutting boards, including one for fruits and vegetables and one for meat, can help prevent cross-contamination and make meal preparation easier.

Knives: a good set of knives, including a chef's knife and a paring knife, can help you prepare ingredients quickly and easily.

Pots and pans: a variety of pots and pans, including a large saucepan, a Dutch oven, and a frying pan, can be used for a variety of cooking methods, such as boiling, braising, and frying.

Measuring cups and spoons: having a set of measuring cups and spoons can ensure that you use the correct amounts of ingredients in your recipes.

Blender: a blender is essential for blending ingredients, such as soups and smoothies, to make them easier to digest.

Slow cooker: a slow cooker is a convenient and easy way to cook meals, as it requires minimal effort and allows you to prepare meals in advance.

By having these essential kitchen tools on hand, you can prepare meals that are not only delicious, but also supportive of a no gallbladder diet. The No Gallbladder Diet Cookbook provides a variety of recipes that make use of these essential kitchen tools to make meal preparation easy and enjoyable.

Explanation of how to select and store ingredients

Ingredients are the building blocks of any dish, and choosing the right ones is key to the success of a recipe. When selecting ingredients, it is important to consider their freshness, quality, and flavor. Here are some tips on how to choose and store ingredients to ensure the best results:

Freshness: Look for ingredients that are in-season and look vibrant and crisp. For example, select ripe tomatoes in the summer, and leafy greens in the fall. Avoid produce that is wilted or has discoloration.

Quality: Choose ingredients that are free of bruises, blemishes, and mold. These imperfections can affect the flavor and texture of the dish.

Flavor: Select ingredients that have a strong, distinct flavor. For example, choose pungent garlic over milder varieties, and opt for sharp cheddar cheese over bland American cheese.

Once you have selected the best ingredients, it is important to store them properly to ensure they stay fresh. Here are some tips for storing ingredients:

Fruits and Vegetables: Store fresh fruits and vegetables in the refrigerator in their original packaging or in airtight containers. Some fruits and vegetables, such as tomatoes and avocados, should not be refrigerated until they are ripe.

Meat and Poultry: Store raw meat and poultry in the refrigerator on the bottom shelf to prevent cross-contamination. Cooked meat should be stored in airtight containers and consumed within three to four days.

Dairy Products: Store dairy products, such as milk and cheese, in the refrigerator. Make sure to check expiration dates and discard any dairy products that have gone bad.

Dry Ingredients: Store dry ingredients, such as flour and sugar, in airtight containers and in a cool, dry place. This will prevent them from becoming contaminated by moisture, insects, or other pests.

By following these tips, you can ensure that you have the best ingredients to make delicious, flavorful dishes.

Foods NOT Allowed in No Gallbladder Diet

The gallbladder is an organ that stores and releases bile, a digestive juice that helps break down fats in the small intestine. If you have had your gallbladder removed, you may experience digestive difficulties, such as abdominal pain and diarrhea, when consuming certain foods. To reduce these symptoms, it is important to follow a no gallbladder diet that avoids certain foods.

Here is a list of foods that are not allowed in a no gallbladder diet:

Fried and greasy foods: Fried and greasy foods, such as French fries, fried chicken, and hamburgers, are difficult to digest for people without a gallbladder. These foods can cause abdominal pain, bloating, and diarrhea.

High-fat dairy products: High-fat dairy products, such as whole milk, cheese, and ice cream, can be difficult to digest without a gallbladder. It is best to choose low-fat or non-fat dairy products instead.

Fatty meats: Fatty meats, such as pork, beef, and lamb, should be avoided on a no gallbladder diet. These meats can cause digestive problems, such as bloating and abdominal pain.

Processed and high-fat snacks: Processed and high-fat snacks, such as chips, crackers, and candy, should be avoided on a no gallbladder diet. These foods can cause digestive problems, such as bloating and diarrhea.

Full-fat salad dressings: Full-fat salad dressings, such as ranch and blue cheese, should be avoided on a no gallbladder diet. These dressings are high in fat and can cause digestive problems, such as bloating and abdominal pain.

Butter and margarine: Butter and margarine are high in fat and should be avoided on a no gallbladder diet. These products can cause digestive problems, such as bloating and diarrhea.

By avoiding these foods, you can reduce your risk of digestive problems and improve your overall health. It is important to talk to your doctor or dietitian before making any changes to your diet, especially if you have any underlying health conditions.

Foods allowed with moderation in No Gallbladder Diet

While a no gallbladder diet typically restricts certain foods, there are still many delicious and nutritious foods that can be consumed in moderation. It is important to listen to your body and pay attention to how different foods affect your digestion.

Here is a list of foods that are allowed with moderation in a no gallbladder diet:

Low-fat dairy products: Low-fat dairy products, such as skim milk, low-fat yogurt, and non-fat cheese, are a good source of calcium and protein. These foods can be consumed in moderation without causing digestive problems.

Lean proteins: Lean proteins, such as chicken, fish, and turkey, are a good source of nutrition and can be consumed in moderation without causing digestive problems.

Whole grains: Whole grains, such as brown rice, whole wheat bread, and oatmeal, are a good source of fiber and nutrients. These foods can be consumed in moderation without causing digestive problems.

It is important to keep portion sizes in mind and to eat slowly to allow for proper digestion. It is also a good idea to avoid eating large meals and to eat smaller, more frequent meals instead. By consuming foods with moderation, you can improve your digestion and maintain a healthy, balanced diet.

Permitted and recommended foods in No Gallbladder Diet

After having your gallbladder removed, it can be challenging to know what foods are safe to eat and which foods to avoid. A no gallbladder diet focuses on eating foods that are easy to digest and that do not cause digestive problems.

Here is a list of permitted and recommended foods in a no gallbladder diet:

Lean proteins: Lean proteins, such as chicken, fish, and turkey, are a good source of nutrition and are recommended for people without a gallbladder. These proteins are easy to digest and do not cause digestive problems.

Fruits and vegetables: Fruits and vegetables are a good source of fiber, vitamins, and minerals. It is best to choose fresh produce and limit the consumption of processed or canned fruits and vegetables.

Nuts and seeds: Nuts and seeds, such as almonds, sunflower seeds, and pumpkin seeds, are a good source of healthy fats, fiber, and protein. These foods are recommended for people without a gallbladder as they are easy to digest and do not cause digestive problems.

Olive oil: Olive oil is a healthy fat that can be used in cooking and as a salad dressing. Olive oil is recommended for people without a gallbladder as it is easy to digest and does not cause digestive problems.

It is important to talk to your doctor or dietitian before making any changes to your diet, especially if you have any underlying health conditions. By incorporating these permitted and recommended foods into your no gallbladder diet, you can improve your digestion, maintain a healthy, balanced diet, and reduce your risk of digestive problems.

Warnings

A no gallbladder diet is designed to help people who have had their gallbladder removed to avoid digestive problems and maintain a healthy, balanced diet. However, there are several warnings that should be kept in mind when following this type of diet.

Consult a healthcare professional: Before making any changes to your diet, it is important to consult with a healthcare professional, such as a doctor or dietitian. They can provide personalized recommendations and help you understand any potential risks or side effects of following a no gallbladder diet.

Avoid high-fat foods: High-fat foods can be difficult to digest for people without a gallbladder, and can cause digestive problems, such as bloating, gas, and diarrhea. It is important to avoid high-fat foods and to limit the amount of fat in your diet.

Limit processed and junk foods: Processed and junk foods, such as fast food and snack foods, are high in unhealthy fats, salt, and sugar. These foods can cause digestive problems and should be limited or avoided on a no gallbladder diet.

Limit alcohol and caffeine: Alcohol and caffeine can cause digestive problems, such as bloating, gas, and diarrhea. It is important to limit your consumption of these beverages and to drink plenty of water instead.

Pay attention to portion sizes: Eating large portions can be difficult to digest for people without a gallbladder and can cause digestive problems. It is important to pay attention to portion sizes and to eat smaller, more frequent meals instead.

Listen to your body: Every person is different and may react differently to different foods. It is important to listen to your body and pay attention to how different foods affect your digestion. If you experience digestive problems, such as bloating, gas, or diarrhea, it may be necessary to avoid certain foods or to adjust your diet.

By following these warnings, you can reduce your risk of digestive problems and maintain a healthy, balanced no gallbladder diet. It is also important to talk to your doctor or dietitian if you have any concerns or questions about your diet.

Breakfast Recipes

Scrambled Eggs with Spinach and Tomatoes

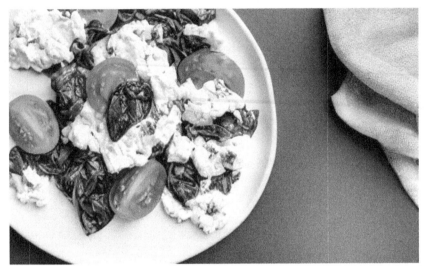

Preparation Time: 5 minutes | Cooking Time: 10 minutes | Serving Size: 2 people

Ingredients:

4 large eggs

2 cups fresh spinach

1 large tomato, diced

1/4 teaspoon salt

1/4 teaspoon black pepper

1 tablespoon olive oil

1/4 cup grated cheese (optional)

Instructions:

In a large bowl, whisk the eggs, salt, and pepper together.

Heat a non-stick pan over medium heat and add the olive oil.

Once the pan is hot, add the diced tomato and sauté for 2-3 minutes.

Add the spinach to the pan and cook until wilted, about 2-3 minutes.

Pour the beaten eggs into the pan and stir gently until the eggs are cooked through, about 3-5 minutes.

If using cheese, sprinkle it on top of the eggs and cook until melted.

Serve immediately and enjoy!

Nutrition Facts (per serving):

Calories: 231 | Fat: 18g | Protein: 14g | Carbohydrates: 7g | Fiber: 2g | Sugar: 3g | Sodium: 473mg.

Whole Grain Toast with Almond Butter and Banana

Preparation Time: 5 minutes | Cooking Time: 2 minutes | Serving Size: 1 person

Ingredients:
2 slices of whole grain bread
2 tablespoons almond butter
1 medium banana, sliced

Instructions:
Toast the bread slices until golden brown.
Spread 1 tablespoon of almond butter on each slice of toast.
Arrange the sliced bananas on top of the almond butter.
Serve immediately and enjoy!

Nutrition Facts (per serving):
Calories: 396 | Fat: 22g | Protein: 11g | Carbohydrates: 44g | Fiber: 8g | Sugar: 14g | Sodium: 208mg

Oatmeal with Berries and Almonds

Preparation Time: 2 minutes | Cooking Time: 5 minutes | Serving Size: 1 person

Ingredients:
1/2 cup old-fashioned oats
1 cup water or almond milk
1/4 teaspoon salt
1/2 cup mixed berries (fresh or frozen)
2 tablespoons almonds, chopped
1 tablespoon honey (optional)

Instructions:
In a small saucepan, bring water or almond milk and salt to a boil.
Stir in the oats and reduce heat to low. Cook, stirring occasionally, for 5 minutes or until the oats are tender and the mixture is thick.
Remove from heat and stir in the mixed berries and almonds.
If desired, drizzle with honey and serve immediately.

Nutrition Facts (per serving):
Calories: 365 | Fat: 12g | Protein: 11g | Carbohydrates: 56g | Fiber: 9g | Sugar: 18g | Sodium: 336mg

Greek Yogurt with Honey and Granola

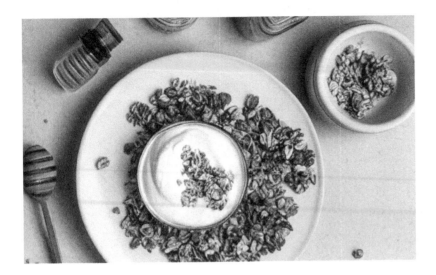

Preparation Time: 2 minutes | Cooking Time: 0 minutes | Serving Size: 1 person

Ingredients:
1 cup plain Greek yogurt
2 tablespoons granola
1 tablespoon honey (optional)

Instructions:
In a bowl, spoon the Greek yogurt.
Sprinkle the granola on top of the yogurt.
If desired, drizzle with honey and serve immediately.

Nutrition Facts (per serving):
Calories: 187 | Fat: 6g | Protein: 18g | Carbohydrates: 19g | Fiber: 1g | Sugar: 13g | Sodium: 80mg.

Vegetable Frittata with Potato and Bell Peppers

Preparation Time: 10 minutes | Cooking Time: 20 minutes | Serving Size: 4 people

Ingredients:
6 large eggs
1 medium potato, peeled and diced
1 bell pepper, diced
1/4 cup onion, diced
1 tablespoon olive oil
1/4 teaspoon salt

1/4 teaspoon black pepper
1/4 cup grated cheese (optional)

Instructions:

In a large bowl, whisk the eggs, salt, and pepper together.

In a large non-stick oven-safe skillet, heat the olive oil over medium heat.

Add the potato, bell pepper, and onion to the skillet and cook until the vegetables are tender, about 10 minutes.

Pour the beaten eggs into the skillet and stir gently to distribute the vegetables evenly.

If using cheese, sprinkle it on top of the eggs.

Place the skillet in the oven and bake for 10 minutes or until the frittata is set and lightly browned.

Serve immediately and enjoy!

Nutrition Facts (per serving):

Calories: 157 | Fat: 11g | Protein: 11g | Carbohydrates: 8g | Fiber: 1g | Sugar: 2g | Sodium: 375mg.

Smoked Salmon and Cream Cheese Bagel

Preparation Time: 5 minutes | Cooking Time: 0 minutes | Serving Size: 1 person

Ingredients:

1 plain bagel, toasted

2 tablespoons cream cheese

2 ounces smoked salmon

1 tablespoon capers (optional)

1/2 lemon, sliced (optional)

Instructions:

Toast the bagel to your desired level of crispiness.

Spread cream cheese evenly on the toasted bagel.

Layer the smoked salmon on top of the cream cheese.

If desired, add capers and a squeeze of lemon juice.

Serve immediately and enjoy!

Nutrition Facts (per serving):

Calories: 366 | Fat: 16g | Protein: 20g | Carbohydrates: 36g | Fiber: 2g | Sugar: 3g | Sodium: 964mg.

Baked Sweet Potato with Cinnamon and Maple Syrup

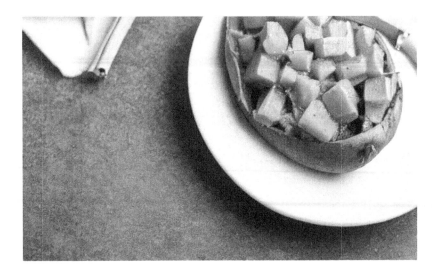

Preparation Time: 5 minutes | Cooking Time: 40 minutes | Serving Size: 1 person

Ingredients:
1 large sweet potato
1 teaspoon cinnamon
1 tablespoon pure maple syrup
1 tablespoon unsalted butter (optional)

Instructions:
Preheat the oven to 400°F (204°C).
Rinse and pat dry the sweet potato.
Pierce the sweet potato several times with a fork.
Place the sweet potato on a baking sheet and bake for 40 minutes, or until soft and tender.
Remove from oven and let cool for a few minutes.
Cut open the sweet potato and add cinnamon, maple syrup, and butter (if using).
Serve hot and enjoy!

Nutrition Facts (per serving):
Calories: 207 | Fat: 2g | Protein: 3g | Carbohydrates: 49g | Fiber: 7g | Sugar: 17g | Sodium: 20mg.

Quinoa Bowl with Fresh Fruits and Nuts

Preparation Time: 10 minutes | Cooking Time: 20 minutes | Serving Size: 1 person

Ingredients:
½ cup quinoa
1 cup water
½ teaspoon salt
1 cup mixed fresh fruits (e.g. berries, sliced banana, diced mango)
2 tablespoons mixed nuts (e.g. almonds, walnuts, pecans)
1 tablespoon honey
1 tablespoon lemon juice

Instructions:
Rinse the quinoa and place it in a saucepan with the water and salt.
Bring to a boil, then reduce the heat to low and let simmer, covered, for about 20 minutes, or until the quinoa has absorbed all the water and is tender.
Remove from heat and let cool for a few minutes.
In a separate bowl, mix together the mixed fruits, mixed nuts, honey, and lemon juice.
Place the quinoa in a serving bowl and top with the fruit and nut mixture.
Serve and enjoy!

Nutrition Facts (per serving):
Calories: 437 | Fat: 16g | Protein: 12g | Carbohydrates: 67g | Fiber: 7g | Sugar: 26g | Sodium: 735mg.

Egg and Vegetable Muffins

Preparation Time: 10 minutes | Cooking Time: 20 minutes | Serving Size: 6 muffins

Ingredients:
6 large eggs
½ cup diced bell pepper
½ cup diced onion
½ cup diced mushrooms
½ cup grated cheddar cheese
Salt and pepper to taste

Instructions:
Preheat the oven to 375°F. Line a muffin tin with 6 muffin liners.
In a large bowl, whisk the eggs.

Stir in the bell pepper, onion, mushrooms, grated cheese, salt, and pepper.

Divide the mixture evenly among the 6 muffin liners.

Bake for 20 minutes, or until the muffins are set and lightly golden.

Remove from the oven and let cool for a few minutes before serving.

Nutrition Facts (per muffin):
Calories: 109 | Fat: 8g | Protein: 9g | Carbohydrates: 3g | Fiber: 1g | Sugar: 2g | Sodium: 191mg.

Smoothie Bowl with Berries, Banana and Almond Milk

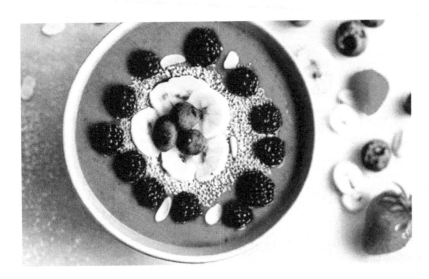

Preparation Time: 5 minutes | Cooking Time: 0 minutes | Serving Size: 1 bowl

Ingredients:
1 banana
1 cup mixed berries (strawberries, blueberries, raspberries)
1/2 cup almond milk
1 tbsp honey
1 tbsp almond butter
1 tsp vanilla extract
2 tbsp granola (for topping)
Fresh berries and sliced banana (for topping)

Instructions:
Add the banana, mixed berries, almond milk, honey, almond butter, and vanilla extract to a blender.

Blend until smooth and creamy.

Pour the smoothie into a bowl.

Top with granola, fresh berries, and sliced banana.

Serve immediately and enjoy.

Nutrition Facts (per serving):
Calories: 361 | Fat: 14g | Protein: 7g | Carbohydrates: 57g | Fiber: 10g | Sugar: 36g | Sodium: 111mg.

Baked Egg and Avocado Boat

Preparation Time: 5 minutes | Cooking Time: 15 minutes | Serving Size: 1 avocado boat

Ingredients:
1 ripe avocado
1 large egg
Salt and pepper to taste
1 tsp olive oil
Fresh herbs (such as cilantro or parsley), for garnish (optional)

Instructions:
Preheat the oven to 400°F.
Cut the avocado in half, lengthwise, and remove the pit.
Place the avocado halves in a baking dish.
Crack an egg into each avocado half, being careful not to break the yolk.
Drizzle olive oil over the egg and avocado.
Season with salt and pepper.
Bake for 15 minutes, or until the egg is set to your liking.
Serve immediately, garnished with fresh herbs, if desired.

Nutrition Facts (per serving):
Calories: 235 | Fat: 21g | Protein: 7g | Carbohydrates: 11g | Fiber: 9g | Sugar: 2g | Sodium: 123mg.

Sweet Potato Hash with Eggs and Turkey Bacon

Preparation Time: 10 minutes | Cooking Time: 20 minutes | Servings: 2

Ingredients:
2 medium sweet potatoes, peeled and diced
4 strips of turkey bacon, diced
2 large eggs
1 tablespoon of olive oil
Salt and pepper to taste
Fresh herbs (optional)

Instructions:
Heat a large skillet over medium heat and add olive oil.
Add diced sweet potatoes and season with salt and pepper. Cook for 10-12 minutes or until tender.
Add diced turkey bacon to the skillet and cook until crispy, about 5 minutes.
In a separate skillet, scramble the eggs and set aside.
Mix the cooked eggs with the sweet potato and turkey bacon mixture.
Serve in a large bowl and sprinkle with fresh herbs if desired.

Nutrition Facts (per serving)
Total Calories: 301 | Total Fat: 15.7g | Saturated Fat: 3.8g | Total Carbohydrates: 31.1g | Fiber: 4.8g | Protein: 12.6g | Cholesterol: 186mg | Sodium: 632mg

Pancakes with Banana and Blueberries

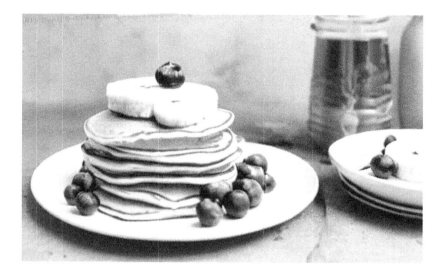

Preparation Time: 10 minutes | Cooking Time: 15 minutes | Serving Size: 2

Ingredients:
1 ripe banana, mashed
1 cup whole grain flour
1 tsp baking powder
1 egg
1 cup unsweetened almond milk
1 tsp vanilla extract
1/4 tsp salt
1/2 cup blueberries
1 tsp coconut oil or non-stick spray
1 tbsp maple syrup (optional)

Instructions:
In a medium mixing bowl, mix together the flour, baking powder and salt.

In a separate bowl, whisk the egg and add in the mashed banana, almond milk and vanilla extract. Stir until well combined.

Pour the wet mixture into the dry mixture and stir until just combined. Gently fold in the blueberries.

Heat the coconut oil or non-stick spray in a large non-stick pan over medium heat.

Using a 1/4 cup measuring cup, pour the batter into the pan and cook until bubbles form on the surface, about 2-3 minutes. Flip and cook until the other side is golden brown, about 1-2 minutes.

Repeat with the remaining batter.

Serve the pancakes with a drizzle of maple syrup and additional blueberries, if desired.

Nutrition Facts (per serving):
Calories: 300 | Fat: 7g | Saturated Fat: 1.5g | Cholesterol: 95mg | Sodium: 430mg | Carbohydrates: 52g | Fiber: 4g | Sugar: 15g | Protein: 10g

Baked Oatmeal with Apples and Cinnamon

Preparation Time: 10 minutes | Cooking Time: 40 minutes | Serves: 4

Ingredients:
2 cups old-fashioned oats
1 tsp baking powder
1 tsp cinnamon
1/4 tsp salt
2 large eggs
1 cup almond milk
1/4 cup maple syrup
2 tsp vanilla extract
2 medium apples, peeled and diced
1/2 cup chopped walnuts (optional)

Instructions:
Preheat oven to 375°F (190°C). Grease an 8x8 inch baking dish.

In a large mixing bowl, combine oats, baking powder, cinnamon, and salt.

In a separate bowl, beat the eggs, almond milk, maple syrup, and vanilla extract until well combined.

Add the egg mixture to the oat mixture, stirring until well combined.

Fold in the diced apples and walnuts (if using).

Pour the oat mixture into the prepared baking dish.

Bake for 35 to 40 minutes or until the top is golden brown and the oatmeal is set.

Let cool for a few minutes before serving. Enjoy!

Nutrition Facts (per serving):
Calories: 333 | Fat: 12g | Saturated Fat: 2g | Cholesterol: 77mg | Sodium: 251mg | Carbohydrates: 51g | Fiber: 6g | Sugar: 25g | Protein: 11g

Breakfast Wrap with Scrambled Eggs and Veggies

Preparation time: 10 minutes | Cooking time: 10 minutes | Serving size: 1 wrap

Ingredients:
1 large whole grain wrap
2 large eggs
1/4 cup of chopped vegetables (bell peppers, onion, mushrooms, etc.)
1 tablespoon of olive oil
Salt and pepper to taste

Instructions:
In a medium-sized pan, heat the olive oil over medium heat.
Add the chopped vegetables and cook until they are tender, around 5 minutes.
In a small bowl, whisk the eggs and season with salt and pepper.
Pour the eggs into the pan with the cooked vegetables and scramble until fully cooked, around 3-5 minutes.
Warm the wrap in a pan or the microwave.
Place the scrambled eggs and veggies in the center of the wrap, fold in the sides and roll up the wrap tightly.

Nutrition Facts per serving (1 wrap)
Calories: 255 | Fat: 15g | Protein: 14g | Carbs: 16g | Fiber: 3g | Sodium: 330mg

Whole Grain Toast with Peanut Butter and Jelly

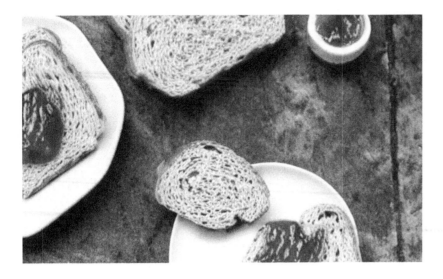

Preparation Time: 5 minutes | Cooking Time: 0 minutes | Serving: 1

Ingredients:

2 slices of whole grain bread

2 tablespoons of peanut butter

2 tablespoons of jelly or fruit spread

Optional: sliced bananas, chopped nuts or honey for toppings

Instructions:

Toast the bread slices until they are golden and crispy.

Spread a generous amount of peanut butter on each slice of toast.

Top each slice with jelly or fruit spread.

If desired, add sliced bananas, chopped nuts, or drizzle with honey.

Serve immediately and enjoy!

Nutrition Facts per serving (based on 2 slices of whole grain bread, 2 tablespoons of peanut butter, and 2 tablespoons of jelly or fruit spread):

Calories: 550 | Fat: 24g | Saturated Fat: 4g | Cholesterol: 0mg | Sodium: 500mg | Carbohydrates: 70g | Fiber: 8g | Sugar: 28g | Protein: 16g

Chia Pudding with Fresh Fruits and Coconut Milk

Preparation time: 5 minutes | Cooking time: 2 hours (chilling time) | Serving size: 2

Ingredients:
1 cup coconut milk
1/2 cup chia seeds
1 tbsp maple syrup
1 tsp vanilla extract
1 cup mixed fresh fruits (e.g., berries, mango, kiwi)
1/4 cup shredded coconut, optional
2 tbsp sliced almonds, optional

Instructions:
In a medium bowl, whisk together coconut milk, chia seeds, maple syrup, and vanilla extract.
Cover the bowl and refrigerate for 2 hours or until the mixture has thickened into a pudding-like consistency.
Divide the chia pudding into two serving bowls.
Top each bowl with mixed fruits, shredded coconut, and sliced almonds.
Serve and enjoy.

Nutrition facts (per serving)
Calories: 280 | Total Fat: 21g | Saturated Fat: 15g | Cholesterol: 0mg | Sodium: 50mg | Total Carbohydrates: 21g | Dietary Fiber: 11g | Sugar: 8g | Protein: 6g |

Granola with Yogurt and Fresh Berries

Preparation time: 10 minutes | Cooking time: 0 minutes | Serving size: 1 bowl

Ingredients:
1/2 cup plain Greek yogurt
1/4 cup granola
1/2 cup mixed berries (strawberries, blueberries, raspberries)
1 tbsp honey
1 tbsp chopped almonds (optional)

Instructions:
In a bowl, add the Greek yogurt.
Top with granola and mixed berries.
Drizzle with honey and sprinkle with chopped almonds, if using.
Serve immediately.

Nutrition facts (per serving):
Calories: 269 | Total Fat: 8g | Saturated Fat: 2g | Cholesterol: 5mg | Sodium: 96mg | Total Carbohydrates: 40g | Dietary Fiber: 3g | Sugars: 25g | Protein: 16g

Breakfast Salad with Egg, Avocado, and Tomato

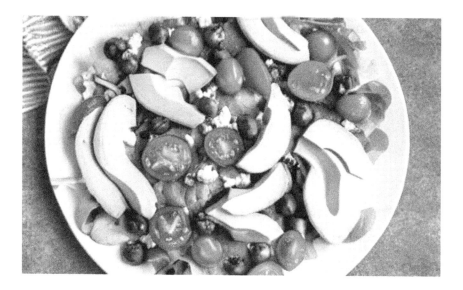

Preparation Time: 10 minutes | Cooking Time: 10 minutes | Serves: 2

Ingredients:

2 large eggs
1 avocado, pitted and diced
1 large tomato, diced
2 cups mixed greens
Salt and pepper, to taste
Olive oil, for cooking
Optional: balsamic vinegar, for dressing

Instructions:

Heat a small non-stick pan over medium heat and add a drizzle of olive oil.
Crack the eggs into the pan and cook until the whites are set and the yolks are still runny, about 3-4 minutes. Season with salt and pepper.
In a large bowl, combine the mixed greens, avocado, and tomato.
Place the eggs on top of the salad and season with additional salt and pepper, if desired.
Optional: drizzle with balsamic vinegar, if desired. Serve immediately.

Nutrition Facts (per serving)

Calories: 325 | Total Fat: 27g | Saturated Fat: 7g | Cholesterol: 186mg | Sodium: 160mg | Total Carbohydrates: 14g | Dietary Fiber: 8g | Sugar: 4g | Protein: 14g

Whole Grain Waffles with Fruit and Honey Syrup

Preparation time: 10 minutes | Cooking time: 10 minutes | Serving size: 2-4

Ingredients:
1 and 1/2 cups whole grain flour
2 teaspoons baking powder
1/2 teaspoon salt
2 large eggs
1 and 1/2 cups almond milk
2 tablespoons melted butter
1 teaspoon vanilla extract
Your choice of fresh fruit (e.g. berries, sliced bananas, peaches)
Honey syrup (equal parts honey and warm water)

Instructions:
In a large mixing bowl, whisk together the flour, baking powder, and salt.
In another bowl, beat the eggs and then mix in the almond milk, melted butter, and vanilla extract.
Pour the wet mixture into the dry mixture and stir until just combined.
Heat a waffle iron and cook the batter until golden brown and crispy. Repeat until all the batter has been used.
Serve the waffles warm with fresh fruit and drizzled with honey syrup.

Nutrition facts (per serving, based on 4 servings)
Calories: 411| Fat: 18 g | Saturated fat: 9 g | Cholesterol: 143 mg | Sodium: 487 mg | Carbohydrates: 54 g |
Fiber: 7 g | Sugar: 15 g | Protein: 12 g

Snacks and Desserts Recipes

Avocado and Cucumber Bites

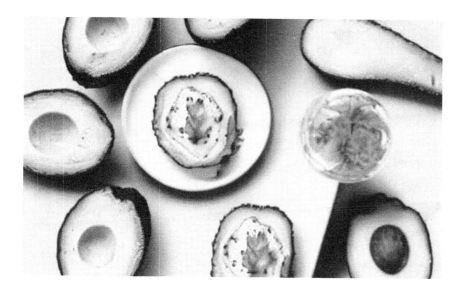

Preparation Time: 10 minutes | Cooking Time: 0 minutes | Serves: 4

Ingredients:
2 ripe avocados, diced
1 cucumber, peeled and diced
2 tbsp. lemon juice
2 tbsp. chopped fresh cilantro
Salt and pepper, to taste
4 whole grain crackers

Instructions:
In a medium bowl, combine the avocado, cucumber, lemon juice, cilantro, salt, and pepper.
Spoon the mixture onto crackers.
Serve immediately and enjoy!

Nutrition Facts per serving (1 bite):
Calories: 80 | Total Fat: 7g | Saturated Fat: 1g | Cholesterol: 0mg | Sodium: 100mg | Total Carbohydrates: 5g | Dietary Fiber: 2g | Total Sugars: 1g | Protein: 1g

Apple and Almond Butter Snack

Preparation Time: 5 minutes | Cooking Time: 0 minutes | Serves: 1

Ingredients:
1 medium apple, sliced
2 tablespoons almond butter
1 teaspoon honey (optional)
1 pinch of cinnamon (optional)

Instructions:
Slice the apple into thin rounds and arrange on a plate.
Spoon the almond butter into a small bowl and warm in the microwave for 20 seconds or until it is runny.
Drizzle the melted almond butter over the apple slices.
If desired, drizzle with honey and sprinkle with cinnamon.
Serve immediately and enjoy!

Nutrition Facts (per serving)
Calories: 280 | Fat: 24 g | Saturated Fat: 2 g | Cholesterol: 0 mg | Sodium: 4 mg | Carbohydrates: 18 g |
Fiber: 5 g | Sugar: 13 g | Protein: 6 g

Baked Sweet Potato Fries

Preparation Time: 10 minutes | Cooking Time: 30 minutes | Serving Size: 4

Ingredients:
2 medium sweet potatoes
2 tablespoons olive oil
1 teaspoon salt
1 teaspoon black pepper
1 teaspoon paprika
1 teaspoon garlic powder

Instructions:
Preheat oven to 400°F (200°C). Line a baking sheet with parchment paper.
Cut the sweet potatoes into 1/4 inch thick fries.
In a large bowl, mix together the sweet potatoes, olive oil, salt, pepper, paprika, and garlic powder.
Transfer the mixture to the lined baking sheet, spreading it out evenly.
Bake for 25-30 minutes, flipping the fries halfway through, until they are golden brown and crispy.
Serve hot and enjoy!

Nutrition Facts (per serving)
Total Calories: 246 | Total Fat: 14g | Saturated Fat: 2g | Cholesterol: 0mg | Sodium: 748mg | Total Carbohydrates: 29g | Dietary Fiber: 4g | Sugar: 6g | Protein: 2g

Zucchini Noodle Salad with Yogurt Dressing

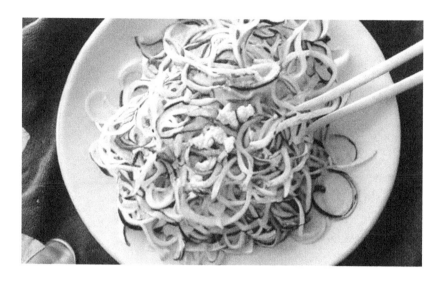

Preparation time: 15 minutes | Cooking time: 0 minutes | Serves: 4

Ingredients:
4 medium zucchinis, spiralized
1 red bell pepper, julienned
1 yellow bell pepper, julienned
1 cup cherry tomatoes, halved
1/2 red onion, thinly sliced
1 cup plain Greek yogurt
2 tablespoons extra-virgin olive oil
2 tablespoons fresh lemon juice
1 teaspoon honey
1/2 teaspoon dried dill
Salt and pepper, to taste

Instructions:
In a large bowl, mix together the spiralized zucchinis, julienned bell peppers, cherry tomatoes, and sliced red onion.
In a small bowl, whisk together the Greek yogurt, olive oil, lemon juice, honey, dried dill, salt, and pepper.
Pour the dressing over the zucchini noodle mixture and gently toss to combine.
Serve chilled and enjoy!

Nutrition Facts (per serving)

Calories: 189 | Total Fat: 14g | Saturated Fat: 2g | Cholesterol: 4mg | Sodium: 106mg | Total Carbohydrates: 16g | Dietary Fiber: 3g | Sugars: 10g | Protein: 8g

Baked Banana Chips with Cinnamon

Preparation Time: 10 minutes | Cooking Time: 40 minutes | Serving Size: 4 servings

Ingredients:
4 ripe bananas
1 tbsp. lemon juice
1 tsp. cinnamon
1 tsp. sugar (optional)

Instructions:
Preheat your oven to 200°F (93°C). Line a baking sheet with parchment paper.
Slice the bananas into rounds, about 1/4 inch thick.
In a small bowl, mix together the lemon juice, cinnamon, and sugar (if using).
Arrange the banana slices on the prepared baking sheet.
Brush the lemon juice mixture over the banana slices.
Bake for 20 minutes, then flip the slices and bake for an additional 20 minutes, or until crispy.
Let cool on the baking sheet for 5 minutes.
Serve as a snack or as a topping for yogurt, oatmeal, or ice cream.

Nutrition Facts (per serving)
Calories: 123 | Fat: 1g | Saturated Fat: 0g | Carbohydrates: 31g | Fiber: 3g | Protein: 2g | Sodium: 1mg | Potassium: 467mg | Sugar: 17g

Roasted Chickpeas with Herbs

Preparation time: 10 minutes | Cooking time: 25 minutes | Serving size: 4

Ingredients:
1 can (15 oz) chickpeas, drained and rinsed
1 tbsp olive oil
1 tsp dried basil
1 tsp dried thyme
1 tsp garlic powder
1 tsp paprika
Salt and pepper, to taste

Instructions:
Preheat oven to 400°F. Line a large baking sheet with parchment paper.
In a bowl, mix together chickpeas, olive oil, basil, thyme, garlic powder, paprika, salt, and pepper.
Spread the chickpeas evenly on the prepared baking sheet.
Bake in the preheated oven for 25 minutes, stirring occasionally, until golden brown and crispy.
Serve warm.

Nutrition facts (per serving)
Calories: 196 | Fat: 8.8g | Saturated Fat: 1.2g | Sodium: 330mg | Carbohydrates: 25g | Fiber: 6.3g | Sugar: 2.6g | Protein: 8g

Fruit Salad with Coconut Milk Yogurt

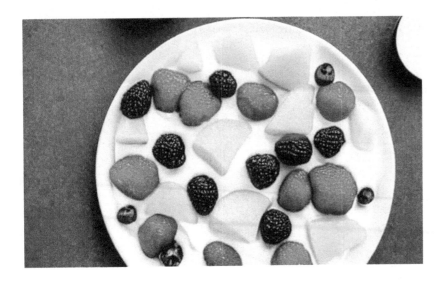

Preparation Time: 10 minutes | Cooking Time: 0 minutes | Serving Size: 4

Ingredients:
4 cups mixed fruit (e.g. strawberries, blueberries, grapes, kiwi, mango, pineapple)
1 cup coconut milk yogurt
1 tablespoon honey
1 teaspoon vanilla extract
1/4 teaspoon cinnamon
Fresh mint leaves, to garnish (optional)

Instructions:
Wash and chop all the fruit into bite-sized pieces.
In a large bowl, mix together the coconut milk yogurt, honey, vanilla extract, and cinnamon.
Add the fruit to the bowl and mix well until all the fruit is coated in the yogurt mixture.
Serve the fruit salad in individual bowls and garnish with fresh mint leaves, if desired.

Nutrition Facts per serving (about 1 cup):
Calories: 183 | Total Fat: 6g | Saturated Fat: 5g | Cholesterol: 3mg | Sodium: 41mg | Total Carbohydrates: 32g | Dietary Fiber: 3g | Sugar: 26g | Protein: 4g

Baked Apple Chips with Cinnamon and Sweetener

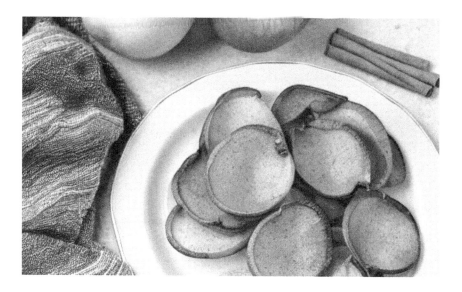

Preparation Time: 10 minutes | Cooking Time: 45 minutes | Serving Size: 4

Ingredients:
4 medium apples (sliced thin)
1 teaspoon ground cinnamon
2 tablespoons of your choice of sweetener (e.g. honey, maple syrup, sugar)

Instructions:
Preheat the oven to 225°F. Line a large baking sheet with parchment paper.
In a bowl, mix together the sweetener and cinnamon.
Arrange the apple slices in a single layer on the prepared baking sheet.
Brush the apple slices with the cinnamon-sweetener mixture.
Bake for 45 minutes or until the edges of the apple slices start to turn golden brown.
Remove from the oven and let cool completely on the baking sheet.
Serve and enjoy!

Nutrition Facts per serving (1/4 of the recipe):
Calories: 70 kcal | Total Fat: 0 g | Sodium: 0 mg | Total Carbohydrates: 18 g | Dietary Fiber: 2 g | Sugar: 14 g | Protein: 1 g

Carrot and Celery Sticks with Hummus

Preparation Time: 10 minutes | Cooking Time: 0 | Serving Size: 4

Ingredients:
4 medium carrots, cut into sticks
4 medium celery stalks, cut into sticks
1 cup of hummus

Instructions:
Wash and cut the carrots and celery stalks into sticks.
Serve the carrot and celery sticks with the hummus in a small bowl for dipping.

Nutrition Facts (per serving)
Calories: 140 | Fat: 10g | Saturated Fat: 1.5g | Cholesterol: 0mg | Sodium: 200mg | Carbohydrates: 11g |
Fiber: 4g | Sugar: 3g | Protein: 4g

Grilled Peach with Almond Butter and Honey

Preparation Time: 5 minutes | Cooking Time: 10 minutes | Servings: 2

Ingredients:
2 ripe peaches, halved and pitted
1/4 cup almond butter
2 tablespoons honey
1/4 teaspoon cinnamon

Instructions:
Heat a grill pan or outdoor grill over medium-high heat.
In a small bowl, mix together almond butter, honey, and cinnamon.
Place peach halves cut side down on the grill and cook for about 5 minutes, or until grill marks appear.
Flip the peaches over and spread the almond butter mixture over the cut side.
Continue cooking for an additional 5 minutes, or until the peaches are tender.
Serve the peaches warm with a drizzle of honey on top, if desired.

Nutrition Facts (per serving):
Calories: 450 | Total Fat: 33g | Saturated Fat: 4g | Cholesterol: 0mg | Sodium: 120mg | Total
Carbohydrates: 42g | Dietary Fiber: 6g | Sugar: 32g | Protein: 9g

Roasted Cauliflower Bites with Lemon and Herbs

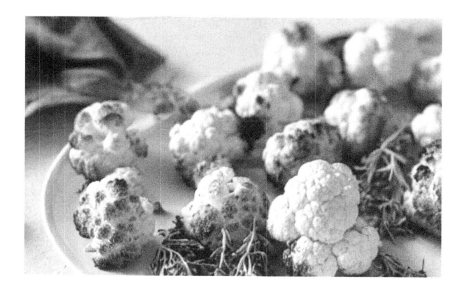

Preparation time: 10 minutes | Cooking time: 25 minutes | Serving size: 4

Ingredients:

1 head of cauliflower, cut into bite-sized florets

2 tablespoons olive oil

1 lemon, zested and juiced

1 teaspoon dried thyme

1 teaspoon dried basil

Salt and pepper, to taste

Instructions:

Preheat oven to 400°F (200°C). Line a baking sheet with parchment paper.

In a large bowl, combine the cauliflower florets, olive oil, lemon zest, lemon juice, thyme, basil, salt, and pepper. Toss to coat the florets evenly.

Spread the mixture evenly on the prepared baking sheet.

Bake for 25 minutes, or until the cauliflower is tender and slightly golden.

Serve immediately.

Nutrition Facts (per serving):

Calories: 140 | Total Fat: 12g | Saturated Fat: 2g | Cholesterol: 0mg | Sodium: 160mg | Total Carbohydrates: 9g | Dietary Fiber: 3g | Sugar: 3g | Protein: 3g

Berry and Yogurt Parfait

Preparation Time: 10 minutes | Cooking Time: 0 minutes | Serving Size: 1

Ingredients:
1 cup mixed berries (strawberries, blueberries, blackberries)
1/2 cup plain Greek yogurt
1 tablespoon honey
1/4 cup granola

Instructions:
Wash and chop the mixed berries if needed.
In a glass or jar, layer the Greek yogurt on the bottom.
Add a layer of mixed berries on top of the yogurt.
Drizzle with honey.
Add another layer of yogurt on top of the berries.
Sprinkle with granola.
Repeat the layering process until the ingredients are used up.
Serve and enjoy immediately.

Nutrition Facts (per serving):
Calories: 250 kcal | Total Fat: 4 g | Saturated Fat: 1 g | Cholesterol: 6 mg | Sodium: 56 mg | Total Carbohydrates: 49 g | Dietary Fiber: 5 g | Sugar: 34 g | Protein: 14 g

Sweet Potato Brownies with Almond Flour

Preparation Time: 15 minutes | Cooking Time: 35 minutes | Servings: 12

Ingredients:
2 medium sweet potatoes, peeled and pureed
2 cups almond flour
1/2 cup unsweetened cocoa powder
1 tsp baking powder
1/2 tsp salt
1/2 cup coconut sugar or brown sugar
3 eggs, lightly beaten
1 tsp vanilla extract
1/2 cup dark chocolate chips (optional)

Instructions:
Preheat oven to 350°F (175°C). Grease a 9x9 inch baking pan and line it with parchment paper.

In a large bowl, whisk together the pureed sweet potatoes, almond flour, cocoa powder, baking powder, salt, and sugar until well combined.

Add the beaten eggs and vanilla extract to the mixture and stir until smooth.

Stir in the chocolate chips, if using.

Pour the batter into the prepared baking pan and bake for 35 minutes or until a toothpick inserted into the center comes out clean.

Let cool completely in the pan before slicing and serving.

Nutrition Facts (per serving)
Calories: 345 | Total Fat: 14g | Saturated Fat: 4g | Cholesterol: 55mg | Sodium: 140mg | Total Carbohydrates: 20g | Dietary Fiber: 4g | Sugars: 12g | Protein: 6g

Banana Oat Cookies with Dark Chocolate Chips

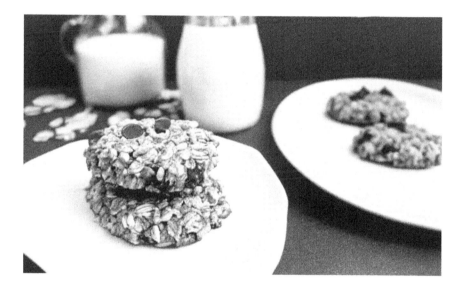

Preparation time: 15 minutes | Cooking time: 12 minutes | Servings: 12 cookies

Ingredients:
2 ripe bananas
1 cup old-fashioned oats
1/2 cup almond flour
1/4 cup coconut sugar
1 tsp baking powder
1 tsp cinnamon
1/4 tsp salt
1 tsp vanilla extract
1/2 cup dark chocolate chips

Instructions:

Preheat your oven to 350°F (175°C) and line a baking sheet with parchment paper.

In a large mixing bowl, mash the bananas using a fork or potato masher.

Add the oats, almond flour, coconut sugar, baking powder, cinnamon, salt, and vanilla extract to the bowl and mix until well combined.

Fold in the dark chocolate chips.

Use a cookie scoop or spoon to form 12 cookie dough balls. Place them on the prepared baking sheet, leaving about 2 inches between each cookie.

Bake for 12 minutes, or until the edges are golden brown and the centers are set.

Remove from oven and allow the cookies to cool for 5 minutes on the baking sheet before transferring to a wire rack to cool completely.

Nutrition Facts per serving (1 cookie):

Calories: 126 | Fat: 6g | Saturated Fat: 3g | Carbohydrates: 18g | Fiber: 2g | Sugar: 9g | Protein: 2g

Baked Cinnamon Sweet Potato Chips

Preparation Time: 15 minutes | Cooking Time: 20 minutes | Serving Size: 4

Ingredients:

4 medium sweet potatoes

1 tbsp. coconut oil, melted

1 tsp. ground cinnamon

1/4 tsp. sea salt

Instructions:

Preheat your oven to 400°F (200°C) and line a baking sheet with parchment paper.

Wash and peel the sweet potatoes and cut them into thin, evenly sized rounds.

In a large mixing bowl, add the sweet potato rounds, melted coconut oil, ground cinnamon, and sea salt. Toss everything together until the sweet potatoes are well coated.

Arrange the sweet potatoes in a single layer on the prepared baking sheet.

Bake for 20-25 minutes or until the sweet potatoes are crispy and golden brown.

Serve immediately and enjoy your Baked Cinnamon Sweet Potato Chips!

Nutrition Facts (per serving):

Calories: 268 | Total Fat: 5g | Saturated Fat: 4g | Cholesterol: 0mg | Total Carbohydrates: 33g | Dietary Fiber: 4g | Total Sugars: 7g | Protein: 2g

Grilled Pineapple with Coconut Sugar and Lime

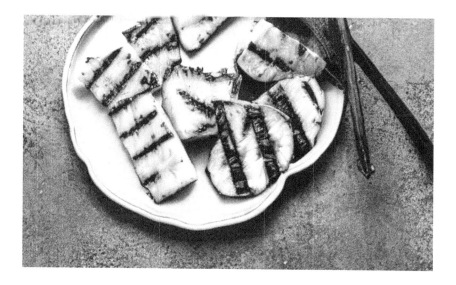

Preparation Time: 10 minutes | Cooking Time: 10 minutes | Serving Size: 4

Ingredients:

1 large pineapple, peeled, cored, and cut into 1/2 inch thick slices
2 tablespoons coconut sugar
1 lime, juiced

Instructions:

Heat a grill pan over medium-high heat.
Arrange the pineapple slices in a single layer on the pan.
Sprinkle the coconut sugar over the pineapple slices.
Grill the pineapple slices for 5 minutes on each side, or until they are golden brown and slightly caramelized.
Remove the pineapple slices from the pan and place them on a serving plate.
Squeeze the lime juice over the grilled pineapple slices.
Serve warm and enjoy!

Nutrition Facts per serving (based on 4 servings):

Calories: 130 | Total Fat: 1g | Saturated Fat: 0g | Trans Fat: 0g | Cholesterol: 0mg | Total Carbohydrates: 33g | Dietary Fiber: 2g | Sugars: 28g | Protein: 1g

Zucchini Bread with Almond Flour

Preparation Time: 15 minutes | Cooking Time: 50-60 minutes | Serving Size: 10 slices

Ingredients:
2 cups almond flour
1 tsp baking powder
1 tsp baking soda
1 tsp cinnamon
1/2 tsp salt
3 eggs
1 cup grated zucchini, squeezed of excess moisture
1/2 cup coconut sugar
1/4 cup melted coconut oil
1 tsp vanilla extract

Instructions:
Preheat the oven to 350°F (180°C).
Grease a 9x5 inch loaf pan with cooking spray.
In a large mixing bowl, combine the almond flour, baking powder, baking soda, cinnamon, and salt.
In another mixing bowl, beat the eggs and mix in the grated zucchini, coconut sugar, melted coconut oil, and vanilla extract.
Combine the wet ingredients with the dry ingredients until just blended.
Pour the batter into the prepared loaf pan and smooth out the top.
Bake for 50-60 minutes or until a toothpick inserted into the center comes out clean.
Allow to cool for 10 minutes in the pan before removing and transferring to a wire rack to cool completely.

Nutrition Facts per slice (1/10 of the loaf):
Calories: 200 | Total Fat: 17g | Saturated Fat: 5g | Trans Fat: 0g | Cholesterol: 60mg | Sodium: 260mg | Total Carbohydrate: 14g | Dietary Fiber: 3g | Total Sugars: 9g | Added Sugars: 6g | Protein: 6g

Avocado Chocolate Mousse with Coconut Milk

Preparation Time: 15 minutes | Cooking Time: 0 minutes | Serving Size: 2

Ingredients:
2 ripe avocados
1/2 cup dark chocolate chips
1/4 cup full-fat coconut milk
2 tbsp honey or maple syrup
1 tsp vanilla extract
Pinch of salt

Instructions:
Melt the dark chocolate chips in a double boiler or in the microwave.
Scoop out the flesh of the avocados into a blender or food processor.
Add melted chocolate, coconut milk, honey or maple syrup, vanilla extract, and salt. Blend until smooth.
Divide the mixture into 2 serving dishes and chill in the refrigerator for 30 minutes.
Serve cold, topped with fresh berries, if desired.

Nutrition Facts per Serving (without toppings):
Calories: 380 | Total Fat: 36 g | Saturated Fat: 20 g | Total Carbohydrates: 22 g | Dietary Fiber: 8 g | Protein: 4 g | Sodium: 20 mg

Baked Cinnamon Apple Chips

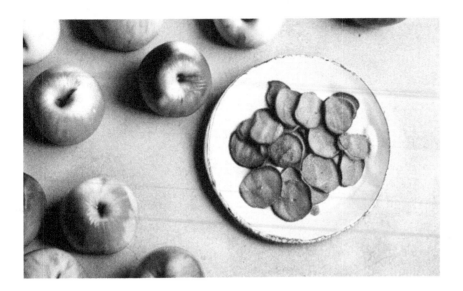

Preparation time: 15 minutes | Cooking time: 1 hour | Serving size: 4

Ingredients:
4 medium apples (such as Gala, Fuji, or Honeycrisp)
1 tbsp ground cinnamon
2 tbsp coconut sugar

Instructions:
Preheat the oven to 200°F (95°C). Line a large baking sheet with parchment paper.

Wash the apples and slice them very thinly using a sharp knife or a mandoline slicer.

In a small bowl, mix the cinnamon and coconut sugar together.

Place the apple slices in a single layer on the prepared baking sheet and sprinkle the cinnamon-sugar mixture over them.

Bake for 1 hour, flipping the apples halfway through the cooking time, until they are dried and crispy.

Allow the apple chips to cool on the baking sheet for a few minutes before serving.

Nutrition facts per serving (4 chips):
Calories: 70 | Total Fat: 0.5g | Saturated Fat: 0g | Sodium: 0mg | Total Carbohydrates: 19g | Dietary Fiber: 2g | Sugar: 14g | Protein: 0.5g

Yogurt and Berry Smoothie Bowl

Preparation Time: 10 minutes | Cooking Time: 0 minutes | Serving Size: 2

Ingredients:

2 cups frozen mixed berries (strawberries, blueberries, raspberries)
1 banana, peeled and frozen
1 cup Greek yogurt
1/2 cup unsweetened almond milk
2 tbsp honey (optional)
Fresh fruit, granola, and nuts for topping (optional)

Instructions:

Add the frozen mixed berries, banana, Greek yogurt, almond milk, and honey (if using) to a blender.
Blend until smooth and creamy, scraping down the sides of the blender as needed.
Pour the smoothie into bowls.
Top with fresh fruit, granola, and nuts, if desired.
Serve immediately and enjoy.

Nutrition Facts (per serving):

Calories: 263 | Fat: 5g | Saturated Fat: 2g | Cholesterol: 15mg | Sodium: 73mg | Carbohydrates: 46g | Fiber: 8g | Sugar: 30g | Protein: 16g.

Main Courses

Slow Cooker Chicken and Vegetables

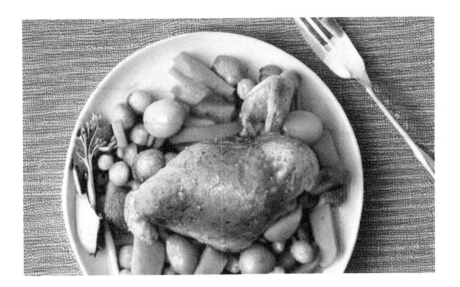

Preparation Time: 15 minutes | Cooking Time: 8 hours | Serving Size: 4-6

Ingredients:
4 boneless, skinless chicken breasts
4 large carrots, peeled and chopped
3 stalks celery, chopped
2 large onions, chopped
4 cloves garlic, minced
1 tsp dried thyme
1 tsp dried rosemary
1 tsp dried basil
Salt and pepper, to taste
2 cups chicken broth

Instructions:
Season chicken breasts with salt, pepper, thyme, rosemary, and basil.
Place chicken in a slow cooker.
Add chopped carrots, celery, onions, and garlic to the slow cooker.
Pour chicken broth over vegetables.
Cook on low heat for 8 hours, or until chicken is cooked through and vegetables are tender.
Serve with your favorite sides.

Nutrition Facts (per serving, based on 6 servings):
Calories: 325 | Total Fat: 5g | Saturated Fat: 1g | Cholesterol: 145mg
Sodium: 890mg | Total Carbohydrates: 15g | Dietary Fiber: 3g | Sugar: 6g
Protein: 59g

Grilled Salmon with Quinoa Salad

Preparation Time | Cooking Time | Serving Size
25 minutes | 25 minutes | 4

Ingredients:
4 salmon fillets (6 ounces each)
1 tablespoon olive oil
Salt and pepper, to taste
2 cups cooked quinoa
1 cup cherry tomatoes, halved
1/2 cup red onion, diced
1/2 cup cucumber, diced
1/4 cup fresh cilantro, chopped
2 tablespoons red wine vinegar
1 tablespoon lemon juice
1 tablespoon honey
Salt and pepper, to taste

Instructions:
Preheat grill to medium-high heat.
Place salmon fillets in a shallow dish and brush both sides with olive oil. Season with salt and pepper.
In a large bowl, combine cooked quinoa, cherry tomatoes, red onion, cucumber, and cilantro.
In a small bowl, whisk together red wine vinegar, lemon juice, honey, and a pinch of salt and pepper. Pour over the quinoa mixture and toss to combine.
Place salmon fillets on the grill and cook for 5-6 minutes per side, or until cooked through.
Serve salmon fillets with quinoa salad.

Nutrition Facts per Serving:
Calories: 385 | Fat: 15g | Saturated Fat: 2g | Cholesterol: 62mg | Sodium: 123mg | Carbohydrates: 33g |
Fiber: 4g | Sugar: 8g | Protein: 29g

Baked Tilapia with Roasted Asparagus

Preparation Time: 15 minutes | Cooking Time: 25 minutes | Serving Size: 4

Ingredients:

4 tilapia fillets (about 6 ounces each)
Salt and pepper, to taste
1/4 teaspoon garlic powder
1/4 teaspoon onion powder
1/4 teaspoon paprika
1/4 teaspoon dried thyme
1 lemon, sliced
2 tablespoons olive oil
1 bunch asparagus, trimmed
1 tablespoon lemon juice

Instructions:

Preheat the oven to 400°F. Line a baking sheet with parchment paper.

Season the tilapia fillets with salt, pepper, garlic powder, onion powder, paprika, and dried thyme.

Arrange the lemon slices on the prepared baking sheet, then place the tilapia fillets on top of the lemon slices.

In a large bowl, combine the asparagus, olive oil, lemon juice, and a pinch of salt and pepper. Toss to coat.

Place the asparagus on the same baking sheet, around the tilapia.

Bake in the preheated oven for 25 minutes or until the fish is opaque and flaky and the asparagus is tender.

Serve the tilapia with the roasted asparagus on the side.

Nutrition Facts per Serving:

Calories: 244 | Total Fat: 14g | Saturated Fat: 2g | Cholesterol: 66mg | Sodium: 331mg | Total Carbohydrates: 7g | Dietary Fiber: 2g | Sugar: 2g | Protein: 25g

Beef Stir-fry with Zucchini Noodles

Preparation Time: 10 minutes | Cooking Time: 20 minutes | Serving Size: 4

Ingredients:

1 pound beef (sirloin or flank steak), sliced into thin strips
4 medium zucchinis, spiralized into noodles
2 tablespoons oil (olive or coconut oil)
3 cloves garlic, minced
1 large onion, sliced
2 bell peppers (red and yellow), sliced
2 tablespoons soy sauce
1 tablespoon honey
1 tablespoon cornstarch
1 teaspoon salt
1 teaspoon black pepper
2 tablespoons chopped fresh herbs (such as basil, cilantro, or parsley)

Instructions:

In a small bowl, whisk together soy sauce, honey, cornstarch, salt, and black pepper.
Heat oil in a large pan over high heat. Add garlic and onion, stir-fry for 2 minutes.
Add beef strips and stir-fry for 3-4 minutes, until browned on all sides.
Add bell peppers, zucchini noodles, and the sauce mixture. Stir-fry for 5 minutes, until the zucchini noodles are tender.
Stir in fresh herbs and serve immediately.

Nutrition Facts (per serving):

Calories: 336 | Fat: 22g | Carbohydrates: 12g | Protein: 26g | Fiber: 3g | Sodium: 1167mg

Turkey and Sweet Potato Shepherd's Pie

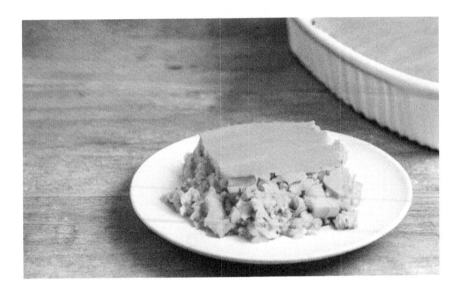

Preparation time: 20 minutes | Cooking time: 1 hour | Serving size: 6-8

Ingredients:
1 lb ground turkey
2 medium sweet potatoes, peeled and diced
1 large onion, diced
2 cloves of garlic, minced
2 medium carrots, diced
2 stalks of celery, diced
1 cup chicken broth
1 cup frozen peas and corn
1 tsp thyme
1 tsp rosemary
Salt and pepper, to taste
2 tbsp olive oil

Instructions:
Preheat oven to 375°F (190°C).

In a large skillet, heat 1 tbsp of olive oil over medium heat. Add the ground turkey and cook until browned, about 10 minutes.

Remove the turkey from the skillet and set aside.

In the same skillet, add the remaining 1 tbsp of olive oil and sauté the onions, garlic, carrots, and celery for 5 minutes, until soft.

Add the cooked ground turkey back to the skillet and add the chicken broth, frozen peas and corn, thyme, rosemary, salt and pepper. Stir to combine and let it simmer for 10 minutes.

While the turkey mixture is simmering, peel and dice the sweet potatoes and steam them until they are soft.

Mash the sweet potatoes with a fork and set aside.

Grease a 9x13 inch baking dish and pour the turkey mixture into the dish.

Spread the mashed sweet potatoes on top of the turkey mixture, covering it evenly.

Bake for 30-40 minutes, or until the top is golden brown.

Serve hot and enjoy!

Nutrition facts (per serving):

Calories: 400 | Fat: 20g | Saturated Fat: 5g | Cholesterol: 70mg | Sodium: 550mg | Carbohydrates: 29g | Fiber: 4g | Sugar: 8g | Protein: 28g

Vegetable and Lentil Soup

Preparation Time: 15 minutes | Cooking Time: 35 minutes | Serving Size: 6

Ingredients:

2 tablespoons of olive oil

1 onion, diced

3 cloves of garlic, minced

2 carrots, peeled and diced

2 celery stalks, diced

1 teaspoon of dried thyme

2 cups of green or brown lentils, rinsed

6 cups of vegetable broth

2 cups of chopped kale

1 cup of diced tomatoes

Salt and pepper, to taste

Instructions:

In a large pot, heat the olive oil over medium heat. Add the onion and cook until softened, about 5 minutes.

Add the garlic, carrots, celery, and thyme. Cook for an additional 5 minutes, stirring occasionally.

Add the lentils, vegetable broth, and kale. Stir to combine.

Bring the soup to a boil, then reduce the heat and let it simmer for 25 minutes, or until the lentils are soft.

Add the diced tomatoes and cook for an additional 5 minutes.

Season with salt and pepper to taste.

Serve the soup hot.

Nutrition Facts (per serving):

Calories: 280 | Total Fat: 7g | Saturated Fat: 1g | Cholesterol: 0mg | Sodium: 750mg | Total Carbohydrates: 40g | Dietary Fiber: 16g | Sugar: 7g | Protein: 16g

Grilled Pork Chops with Mashed Cauliflower

Preparation Time: 20 minutes | Cooking Time: 25 minutes | Serving Size: 4

Ingredients:
4 boneless pork chops
Salt and pepper, to taste
1 tsp garlic powder
1 tsp onion powder
1 tsp dried thyme
1 tsp dried rosemary
1 tsp paprika
1 tbsp olive oil
1 head of cauliflower, chopped
1/2 cup chicken broth
1/4 cup heavy cream
1 tbsp butter
2 garlic cloves, minced

Instructions:
Season the pork chops with salt, pepper, garlic powder, onion powder, thyme, rosemary, and paprika.
Heat olive oil in a large skillet over medium heat.
Add the pork chops to the skillet and cook for 4-5 minutes on each side, or until fully cooked.
While the pork chops are cooking, steam the cauliflower in a saucepan until tender, about 8-10 minutes.
In a separate saucepan, combine the chicken broth, heavy cream, and butter. Heat until the butter is melted and the mixture is hot.
In a food processor or blender, puree the steamed cauliflower with the chicken broth mixture and garlic until smooth.
Serve the pork chops with a side of mashed cauliflower.

Nutrition Facts per serving:
Calories: 435 | Fat: 30g | Saturated Fat: 11g | Cholesterol: 124mg | Sodium: 590mg | Carbohydrates: 8g | Fiber: 3g | Sugar: 3g | Protein: 36g

Chicken and Rice Casserole

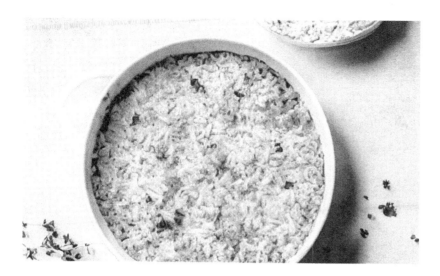

Preparation Time: 20 minutes | Cooking Time: 45 minutes | Serving Size: 6

Ingredients:

1 lb boneless, skinless chicken breasts, cut into 1-inch pieces

1 tbsp olive oil

1 large onion, diced

2 cloves garlic, minced

1 large red bell pepper, diced

2 cups chicken broth

1 cup uncooked white rice

1 tsp salt

1/2 tsp black pepper

1/4 tsp paprika

1/4 tsp dried thyme

1 1/2 cups shredded cheddar cheese

Instructions:

Preheat oven to 375°F.

Heat olive oil in a large skillet over medium heat.

Add chicken to the skillet and cook for about 5 minutes or until browned. Remove chicken from skillet and set aside.

In the same skillet, add onion, garlic, and red bell pepper. Cook until the vegetables are tender, about 5 minutes.

In a large bowl, mix together the cooked chicken, cooked vegetables, chicken broth, uncooked rice, salt, black pepper, paprika, and dried thyme.

Pour the mixture into a 9x13 inch baking dish and cover with aluminum foil.

Bake for 30 minutes.

Remove the foil and sprinkle cheddar cheese on top. Return to the oven and bake for another 15 minutes or until the cheese is melted and bubbly.

Serve hot.

Nutrition Facts per Serving:
Calories: 410 | Fat: 15g | Saturated Fat: 6g | Cholesterol: 95mg | Sodium: 870mg | Carbohydrates: 36g | Fiber: 2g | Sugar: 3g | Protein: 32g

Eggplant Parmesan

Preparation Time: 15 minutes | Cooking Time: 45 minutes | Serving Size: 4

Ingredients:
1 large eggplant, sliced into rounds
2 eggs, beaten
1 cup Italian-seasoned breadcrumbs
1/2 cup all-purpose flour
1 cup marinara sauce
1 cup shredded mozzarella cheese
1/4 cup grated parmesan cheese
Salt and pepper to taste
Olive oil for cooking

Instructions:
Preheat oven to 375°F (190°C).
In a shallow dish, beat the eggs. In another shallow dish, combine the breadcrumbs, flour, salt, and pepper.
Dip the eggplant slices in the beaten eggs, then coat them in the breadcrumb mixture.
In a large skillet, heat the olive oil over medium heat. Cook the eggplant slices until they are browned and crispy, about 3-4 minutes per side.
In a 9x13 inch baking dish, spread 1/2 cup of marinara sauce on the bottom.
Place the eggplant slices on top of the sauce. Spread the remaining sauce over the eggplant.
Sprinkle the mozzarella and parmesan cheese over the sauce.
Bake the eggplant parmesan for 25-30 minutes, or until the cheese is melted and bubbly.
Serve hot.

Nutrition Facts (per serving):
Calories: 400 | Fat: 18g | Saturated Fat: 6g | Cholesterol: 111mg | Sodium: 1020mg | Carbohydrates: 43g | Fiber: 8g | Sugar: 14g | Protein: 22g

Beef and Broccoli Stir-fry

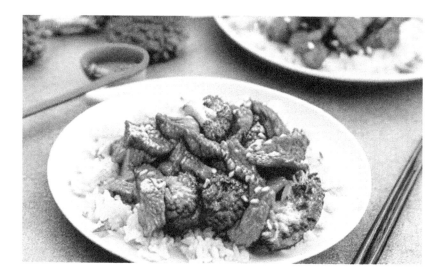

Preparation Time: 10 minutes | Cooking Time: 20 minutes | Serving Size: 4

Ingredients:

1 lb flank steak, sliced thin
3 cups broccoli florets
2 tablespoons oil
2 cloves garlic, minced
2 tablespoons cornstarch
2 tablespoons water
1/4 cup low-sodium soy sauce
2 tablespoons brown sugar
1 tablespoon hoisin sauce
1 teaspoon sesame oil

Instructions:

In a bowl, whisk together the cornstarch and water. Set aside.
In a large wok or frying pan, heat the oil over high heat.
Add the garlic and stir-fry for 30 seconds until fragrant.
Add the sliced steak and stir-fry for 2-3 minutes until browned.
Add the broccoli florets and stir-fry for 2-3 minutes until tender.
In a small bowl, whisk together the soy sauce, brown sugar, hoisin sauce, and sesame oil.
Pour the sauce over the beef and broccoli mixture and stir-fry for 2 minutes until the sauce thickens.
Serve the beef and broccoli stir-fry with rice.

Nutrition Facts per Serving

Total Fat: 17.8g | Saturated Fat: 4.5g | Cholesterol: 57.7mg | Sodium: 597.7mg | Total Carbohydrates: 20.8g | Dietary Fiber: 2.3g | Sugar: 10.7g | Protein: 25.7g

Quinoa Stuffed Bell Peppers

Preparation time: 15 minutes | Cooking time: 40 minutes | Serving size: 4

Ingredients:
4 medium-sized bell peppers
1 cup quinoa, cooked
1 tablespoon olive oil
1 small onion, diced
2 cloves of garlic, minced
1 can diced tomatoes
1 cup corn kernels
1 can of black beans, drained and rinsed
1 teaspoon chili powder
1 teaspoon cumin
Salt and pepper, to taste
1 cup shredded cheddar cheese
Fresh cilantro, for garnish

Instructions:
Preheat oven to 375°F (190°C).
Cut the tops off of the bell peppers and remove the seeds and membranes.
In a large pan over medium heat, heat the olive oil. Add the onion and cook until softened, about 5 minutes.
Add the garlic, diced tomatoes, corn, black beans, chili powder, cumin, salt and pepper to the pan. Cook for 5 minutes until heated through.
Add the cooked quinoa to the pan and mix well to combine.
Fill the bell peppers with the quinoa mixture.
Place the filled bell peppers in a baking dish and bake for 25 minutes.
Sprinkle the shredded cheese on top of the bell peppers and bake for another 15 minutes until cheese is melted and bubbly.
Serve hot, garnished with fresh cilantro.

Nutrition Facts per serving
Calories: 375 | Total Fat: 14g | Saturated Fat: 5g | Cholesterol: 25mg | Sodium: 470mg | Total Carbohydrates: 52g | Dietary Fiber: 10g | Sugars: 10g | Protein: 16g

Grilled Chicken and Mixed Vegetable Skewers

Preparation Time: 25 minutes | Cooking Time: 20 minutes | Serving Size: 4

Ingredients:
4 boneless skinless chicken breasts, cut into 1-inch cubes
2 medium zucchinis, sliced into rounds
1 red bell pepper, cut into 1-inch pieces
1 yellow bell pepper, cut into 1-inch pieces
1 red onion, cut into 1-inch pieces
8 cherry tomatoes
Salt and pepper, to taste
4 tablespoons olive oil
2 tablespoons balsamic vinegar

Instructions:
Preheat the grill to high heat.
In a large bowl, mix together the chicken, zucchini, bell peppers, onion, and cherry tomatoes.
Season with salt and pepper and drizzle with 2 tablespoons of the olive oil and the balsamic vinegar.
Thread the chicken and vegetable mixture onto 8 skewers, alternating between chicken and vegetables.
Brush the skewers with the remaining 2 tablespoons of olive oil.
Place the skewers on the grill and cook for 10-12 minutes on each side, until the chicken is cooked through and the vegetables are slightly charred.
Serve hot.

Nutrition Facts per serving:
Calories: 413 | Total Fat: 26g | Saturated Fat: 4g | Cholesterol: 98mg | Sodium: 116mg | Total Carbohydrates: 12g | Dietary Fiber: 3g | Sugars: 6g | Protein: 33g

Baked Chicken with Sweet Potato Wedges

Preparation Time: 30 minutes | Cooking Time: 35-40 minutes | Serving Size: 4

Ingredients:
4 boneless chicken breasts
4 medium sweet potatoes, peeled and sliced into wedges
2 tablespoons olive oil
Salt and pepper to taste
1 teaspoon paprika
1 teaspoon garlic powder
1 teaspoon dried thyme
1 teaspoon dried rosemary

Instructions:
Preheat oven to 400°F. Line a baking sheet with parchment paper or aluminum foil.
In a large bowl, toss the sweet potato wedges with 1 tablespoon of olive oil, salt, and pepper. Spread them out in a single layer on the prepared baking sheet.
In the same bowl, toss the chicken breasts with the remaining olive oil, paprika, garlic powder, thyme, and rosemary. Place the chicken breasts on the same baking sheet as the sweet potatoes.
Bake in the oven for 35-40 minutes, or until the chicken is cooked through and the sweet potatoes are tender and lightly browned.
Serve the chicken and sweet potatoes together on a plate and enjoy!

Nutrition Facts per serving:
Calories: 375 | Fat: 11.5g | Sodium: 121 mg | Carbohydrates: 43g | Protein: 27g

Turkey and Vegetable Chili

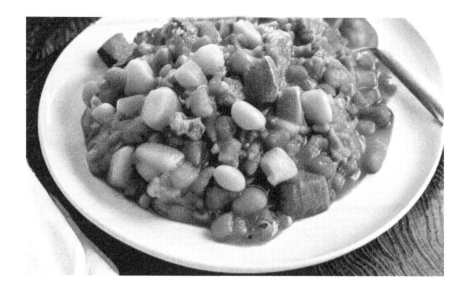

Preparation Time | Cooking Time | Serving Size: 20 minutes | 60 minutes | 6 servings

Ingredients:

1 pound lean ground turkey
1 onion, diced
1 red bell pepper, diced
1 green bell pepper, diced
3 cloves garlic, minced
1 can (14.5 oz) diced tomatoes
2 cups vegetable broth
1 can (15 oz) kidney beans, drained and rinsed
1 can (15 oz) black beans, drained and rinsed
1 can (15 oz) corn, drained
1 tablespoon chili powder
1 teaspoon ground cumin
1/2 teaspoon dried oregano
1/4 teaspoon cayenne pepper
Salt and pepper to taste
Fresh cilantro and shredded cheese for toppings (optional)

Instructions:

In a large pot, cook the ground turkey over medium heat until browned.
Add the diced onion, red and green bell peppers, and minced garlic to the pot and cook until the vegetables are soft and fragrant.
Stir in the diced tomatoes, vegetable broth, kidney beans, black beans, and corn.
Add the chili powder, cumin, oregano, cayenne pepper, salt, and pepper to the pot and stir to combine.
Reduce heat to low, cover, and let the chili simmer for 45-60 minutes, or until the vegetables are tender.
Serve hot, topped with cilantro and shredded cheese if desired.

Nutrition Facts | per serving (1/6 of recipe):
Calories: 284 | Fat: 9g | Cholesterol: 74mg | Sodium: 822mg | Carbohydrates: 27g | Fiber: 9g | Sugar: 5g | Protein: 26g

Baked Cod with Tomato and Olive Relish

Preparation Time: 15 minutes | Cooking Time: 25 minutes | Serving Size: 4

Ingredients:
4 cod fillets, about 6 ounces each
Salt and pepper, to taste
1 tsp. olive oil
1 large tomato, chopped
1/4 cup pitted kalamata olives, chopped
2 tbsp. fresh basil, chopped
1 clove garlic, minced
1 lemon, sliced into wedges

Instructions:
Preheat oven to 400°F.
Season the cod fillets with salt and pepper.
In a large baking dish, arrange the cod fillets.
In a small bowl, mix together the chopped tomato, olives, basil, minced garlic, and olive oil.
Spoon the tomato mixture evenly over the cod fillets.
Place the lemon wedges around the fillets.
Bake for 25 minutes or until the fish is opaque and flakes easily with a fork.
Serve hot with additional lemon wedges, if desired.

Nutrition Facts (Serving Size 1/4 recipe | Servings per recipe 4)
Calories: 151 | Total Fat: 7g | Saturated Fat: 1g | Cholesterol: 47mg | Sodium: 259mg | Total Carbohydrates: 4g | Dietary Fiber: 1g | Sugar: 2g | Protein: 19g

Turkey Meatballs with Spaghetti Squash

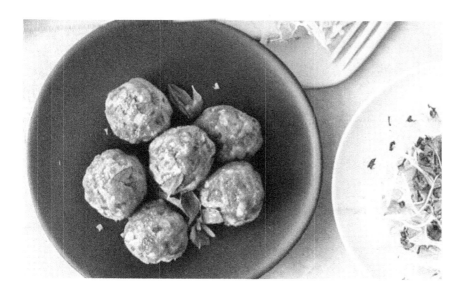

Prep Time: 20 minutes | Cooking Time: 30 minutes | Serving Size: 4

Ingredients:
1 pound ground turkey
1 egg
1/4 cup breadcrumbs
1/4 cup grated Parmesan cheese
1 teaspoon dried basil
1 teaspoon dried oregano
1/2 teaspoon salt
1/4 teaspoon black pepper
1 spaghetti squash
2 tablespoons olive oil
1 teaspoon salt
1/2 teaspoon black pepper
2 tablespoons tomato sauce (optional)

Instructions:
Preheat oven to 400°F (200°C).

In a large bowl, combine ground turkey, egg, breadcrumbs, Parmesan cheese, basil, oregano, salt, and pepper. Mix well to combine.

Shape the mixture into 1-inch meatballs.

Arrange the meatballs on a baking sheet lined with parchment paper. Bake in preheated oven for 25 minutes, or until cooked through.

Meanwhile, cut the spaghetti squash in half lengthwise. Remove the seeds and strings.

Place the spaghetti squash halves, cut-side up, on a baking sheet. Drizzle with olive oil and sprinkle with salt and pepper.

Bake in preheated oven for 30 minutes, or until tender.

Use a fork to scrape the spaghetti squash into long strings. Serve with the turkey meatballs and tomato sauce, if desired.

Nutrition Facts:

Calories: 368 | Total Fat: 22g | Saturated Fat: 6g | Cholesterol: 136mg | Sodium: 711mg | Total Carbohydrates: 13g | Dietary Fiber: 2g | Sugar: 5g | Protein: 31g

Grilled Lamb Chops with Roasted Brussels Sprouts

Preparation Time | Cooking Time | Serving Size
20 minutes | 20 minutes | 4

Ingredients:
4 lamb chops (6 oz each)
2 tablespoons olive oil
1 teaspoon salt
1 teaspoon black pepper
1 teaspoon dried thyme
1 teaspoon dried rosemary
1 teaspoon garlic powder
1 pound brussels sprouts, trimmed and halved

Instructions:
Preheat your grill to medium-high heat.
In a small bowl, mix together the olive oil, salt, black pepper, thyme, rosemary, and garlic powder.
Brush the mixture over the lamb chops and brussels sprouts.
Place the lamb chops and brussels sprouts on the grill, and cook for about 10 minutes on each side, or until the lamb is cooked to your desired level of doneness.
Serve the lamb chops with the roasted brussels sprouts.

Nutrition Facts| Per Serving (Based on 4 servings):
Calories: 434 | Total Fat: 31g | Saturated Fat: 11g | Cholesterol: 111mg | Sodium: 946mg | Total Carbohydrates: 12g | Dietary Fiber: 4g | Sugar: 4g | Protein: 28g

Chicken and Vegetable Bake

Preparation Time. 15 minutes | Cooking Time: 45 minutes | Serving Size: 4

Ingredients:
4 boneless, skinless chicken breasts
2 large carrots, sliced
2 medium zucchinis, sliced
1 red bell pepper, sliced
1 yellow onion, sliced
2 cloves of garlic, minced
1 teaspoon dried basil
1 teaspoon dried thyme
Salt and pepper, to taste
1 tablespoon olive oil
1 cup chicken broth
1/2 cup heavy cream
1 cup shredded mozzarella cheese

Instructions:
Preheat oven to 400°F (200°C).
In a large bowl, mix together sliced carrots, zucchinis, red bell pepper, and onion. Add minced garlic, dried basil, thyme, salt and pepper, and olive oil. Toss to combine.
In a 9x13 inch (23x33 cm) baking dish, place the chicken breasts in the center.
Pour the mixed vegetables around the chicken and pour chicken broth and heavy cream over everything.
Cover the baking dish with aluminum foil and bake for 25 minutes.
After 25 minutes, remove the foil and sprinkle shredded mozzarella cheese over the top.
Bake for another 20 minutes, or until the cheese is melted and the chicken is cooked through (165°F or 74°C internal temperature).
Serve hot.

Nutrition Facts per Serving:
Calories: 460 | Fat: 27g | Saturated Fat: 13g | Cholesterol: 160mg | Sodium: 470mg | Carbohydrates: 13g | Fiber: 3g | Sugar: 6g | Protein: 42g

Beef and Vegetable Skewers with Herb Sauce

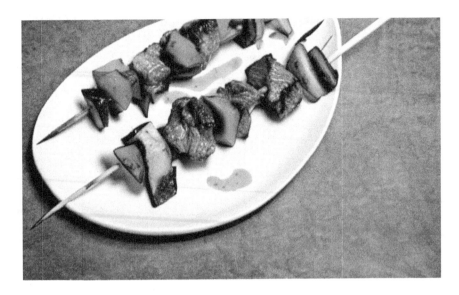

Preparation Time: 15 minutes | Cooking Time: 15 minutes | Serves: 4

Ingredients:

1 1/2 lbs beef sirloin, cut into 1-inch cubes

2 medium bell peppers, cut into 1-inch pieces

1 large red onion, cut into 1-inch pieces

16 cherry tomatoes

8 metal or wooden skewers (if using wooden skewers, soak in water for 30 minutes before using)

Herb Sauce:

1/2 cup plain Greek yogurt

1/4 cup mayonnaise

2 tablespoons fresh lemon juice

1 tablespoon chopped fresh basil

1 tablespoon chopped fresh parsley

1 teaspoon chopped fresh thyme

1 clove garlic, minced

Salt and pepper, to taste

Instructions:

In a small bowl, mix together all of the ingredients for the herb sauce and set aside.

Preheat the grill to high heat.

Alternate beef, bell peppers, red onion, and cherry tomatoes on the skewers.

Place the skewers on the grill and cook for 12-15 minutes, turning occasionally, until the beef is cooked to your desired doneness.

Serve the skewers with the herb sauce on the side for dipping.

Nutrition Facts (per serving):
Calories: 400 | Fat: 26g | Saturated Fat: 8g | Cholesterol: 94mg | Sodium: 240mg | Carbohydrates: 8g | Fiber: 2g | Sugar: 4g | Protein: 33g

Roasted Turkey Breast with Carrots and Parsnips

Preparation Time: 15 minutes | Cooking Time: 60 minutes | Serves: 4-6

Ingredients:
1 large turkey breast (4-5 pounds)
1 1/2 pounds carrots, peeled and cut into 2-inch pieces
1 1/2 pounds parsnips, peeled and cut into 2-inch pieces
4 garlic cloves, minced
2 tablespoons olive oil
1 teaspoon dried thyme
Salt and pepper, to taste
1/4 cup chicken broth

Instructions:
Preheat oven to 400°F. Line a baking sheet with parchment paper.
In a large bowl, combine the carrots, parsnips, garlic, olive oil, thyme, salt, and pepper. Toss to coat the vegetables evenly.
Arrange the vegetables in a single layer on the prepared baking sheet.
Place the turkey breast on top of the vegetables, skin-side up.
Pour the chicken broth over the vegetables and turkey.
Roast for 60 minutes or until the internal temperature of the turkey reaches 165°F.
Let the turkey rest for 10 minutes before slicing and serving with the roasted vegetables.

Nutrition Facts (per serving):
Calories: 450 | Total Fat: 18g | Saturated Fat: 4g | Cholesterol: 140mg | Sodium: 300mg | Total Carbohydrates: 27g | Dietary Fiber: 7g | Sugar: 10g | Protein: 43g

Salad

Grilled Chicken and Avocado Salad

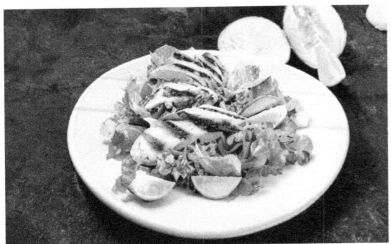

Preparation Time: 15 minutes | Cooking Time: 15 minutes | Serving Size: 4

Ingredients:

4 boneless, skinless chicken breasts

1 tbsp olive oil

Salt and pepper, to taste

2 avocados, diced

2 cups mixed greens

1 cup cherry tomatoes, halved

1/2 red onion, thinly sliced

1/4 cup fresh cilantro leaves

1 lime, juiced

Instructions:

Preheat grill to medium-high heat.

Brush chicken breasts with olive oil and season with salt and pepper.

Place chicken on the grill and cook for 6 to 8 minutes on each side, or until fully cooked through.

Remove chicken from grill and let it rest for a few minutes before slicing.

In a large bowl, combine mixed greens, cherry tomatoes, red onion, cilantro, and lime juice.

Top the salad with sliced chicken and diced avocado.

Serve immediately.

Nutrition Facts (per serving):

Calories: 400 | Fat: 25g | Saturated Fat: 4g | Cholesterol: 95mg | Sodium: 150mg | Carbohydrates: 13g | Fiber: 6g | Sugar: 4g | Protein: 37g

Shrimp and Mango Salad with Lime Dressing

Preparation time: 15 minutes | Cooking time: 5 minutes | Serving size: 4

Ingredients:
1 lb. raw large shrimp, peeled and deveined
2 ripe mangoes, peeled and diced
2 cups of mixed greens
1 red bell pepper, sliced
1 avocado, diced
1/4 cup of red onion, diced
2 limes, juiced
2 tbsp. extra virgin olive oil
Salt and pepper, to taste

Instructions:
Heat a large skillet over medium-high heat. Add the shrimp and cook for 2-3 minutes on each side, or until pink and cooked through. Remove from heat and set aside.
In a large bowl, combine the mangoes, mixed greens, red bell pepper, avocado, and red onion.
In a small bowl, whisk together the lime juice, olive oil, salt, and pepper.
Add the cooked shrimp to the bowl of mixed vegetables and drizzle with the lime dressing. Toss to combine.
Serve immediately, garnished with extra lime wedges and chopped cilantro if desired.

Nutrition Facts (per serving):
Total calories: 312 | Total fat: 23g | Saturated fat: 3g | Cholesterol: 143mg | Sodium: 813mg | Total carbohydrate: 20g | Dietary fiber: 5g | Sugar: 14g | Protein: 15g

Quinoa and Vegetable Salad with Feta Cheese

Preparation Time: 15 minutes | Cooking Time: 20 minutes | Serving Size: 4

Ingredients:
1 cup quinoa
1 red bell pepper, diced
1 yellow bell pepper, diced
1 zucchini, diced
1 cup cherry tomatoes, halved
1/2 cup feta cheese, crumbled
1/4 cup fresh parsley, chopped
1/4 cup fresh mint, chopped
1/4 cup fresh basil, chopped
1/4 cup olive oil
2 tbsp lemon juice
Salt and pepper, to taste

Instructions:
Rinse the quinoa and cook according to package instructions until tender. Let cool to room temperature.
In a large bowl, mix together the cooked quinoa, bell peppers, zucchini, cherry tomatoes, feta cheese, parsley, mint, and basil.
In a small bowl, whisk together the olive oil, lemon juice, salt, and pepper.
Pour the dressing over the quinoa mixture and toss to combine.
Serve chilled or at room temperature.

Nutrition Facts (per serving)
Calories: 350 | Fat: 22g | Protein: 10g | Carbs: 33g | Fiber: 4g | Sodium: 300mg

Greek Salad with Grilled Chicken and Olives

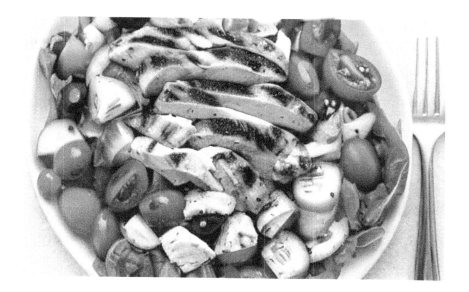

Preparation time: 15 minutes | Cooking time: 15 minutes | Serving size: 4

Ingredients:
4 boneless, skinless chicken breasts
Salt and pepper, to taste
1/4 cup olive oil
4 cups mixed greens
1 large tomato, diced
1 cucumber, peeled and sliced
1 red onion, sliced
1/2 cup kalamata olives
1/2 cup crumbled feta cheese
2 tbsp. red wine vinegar
2 tbsp. lemon juice
1 garlic clove, minced

Instructions:
Preheat your grill to medium-high heat.
Season the chicken breasts with salt and pepper, and brush with 2 tablespoons of olive oil.
Grill the chicken for about 6 to 8 minutes per side or until fully cooked.
In a large bowl, combine the mixed greens, tomato, cucumber, red onion, and olives.
In a small bowl, whisk together the remaining olive oil, red wine vinegar, lemon juice, and minced garlic.
Slice the chicken into thin strips.
Drizzle the dressing over the salad and top with the sliced chicken and feta cheese.
Toss the salad until well combined.
Serve the salad immediately.

Nutrition Facts per serving:
Calories: 450 kcal | Fat: 31g | Saturated Fat: 8g | Cholesterol: 84mg | Sodium: 611mg | Carbohydrates: 14g | Fiber: 3g | Sugar: 4g | Protein: 31g

Arugula and Beet Salad with Walnuts and Goat Cheese

Preparation Time: 15 minutes | Cooking Time: 15 minutes | Serving Size: 4

Ingredients:
4 medium beets, roasted and chopped
5 cups arugula
1/2 cup walnuts, chopped
4 oz. goat cheese, crumbled
2 tbsp. extra-virgin olive oil
2 tbsp. balsamic vinegar
Salt and pepper, to taste

Instructions:
Preheat the oven to 400°F.
Wrap each beet in foil and place them in the oven to roast for about 1 hour, or until they are tender.
Let the beets cool, then peel and chop them into bite-sized pieces.
In a large bowl, combine the arugula, chopped beets, chopped walnuts, and crumbled goat cheese.
In a small bowl, whisk together the olive oil, balsamic vinegar, salt, and pepper to make the dressing.
Drizzle the dressing over the salad and toss to coat evenly.
Serve immediately.

Nutrition Facts per Serving:
Calories: 348 | Fat: 30g | Saturated Fat: 9g | Cholesterol: 25mg | Sodium: 348mg | Carbohydrates: 16g | Fiber: 4g | Sugar: 8g | Protein: 10g

Spinach and Strawberry Salad with Balsamic Vinaigrette

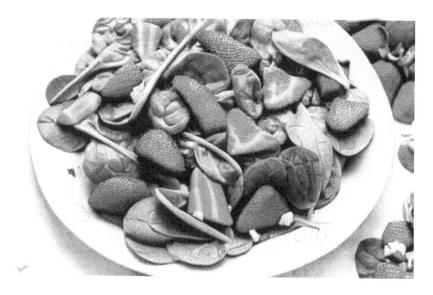

Preparation Time: 20 minutes | Cooking Time: 5 minutes | Serves: 4

Ingredients:

8 cups fresh spinach leaves

2 cups fresh strawberries, hulled and sliced

1/2 cup walnuts, roughly chopped

1/2 cup crumbled goat cheese

2 tablespoons balsamic vinegar

2 tablespoons extra-virgin olive oil

1 teaspoon honey

Salt and pepper, to taste

Instructions:

In a large bowl, combine the spinach leaves, strawberries, walnuts, and goat cheese.

In a small bowl, whisk together the balsamic vinegar, olive oil, honey, salt, and pepper to make the vinaigrette.

Pour the vinaigrette over the salad and gently toss to combine.

Serve the salad immediately and enjoy!

Nutrition Facts (per serving)

Total Fat: 21 g | Saturated Fat: 5 g | Cholesterol: 14 mg | Sodium: 256 mg | Total Carbohydrates: 14 g | Dietary Fiber: 4 g | Sugar: 9 g | Protein: 9 g

Roasted Sweet Potato and Kale Salad with Pomegranate Seeds

Preparation Time | Cooking Time | Serving Size
15 minutes | 45 minutes | 4

Ingredients:
2 large sweet potatoes, peeled and cut into wedges
1 bunch of kale, chopped
1/4 cup olive oil
Salt and pepper, to taste
1/2 cup pomegranate seeds
1/4 cup balsamic vinegar
2 tablespoons honey
2 tablespoons dijon mustard
2 cloves of garlic, minced

Instructions:
Preheat oven to 400°F.
Line a baking sheet with parchment paper and arrange the sweet potato wedges on the sheet.
Drizzle with 2 tablespoons of olive oil and sprinkle with salt and pepper.
Roast the sweet potatoes in the oven for 40-45 minutes, flipping once during cooking, until tender and crispy.
While the sweet potatoes are cooking, make the dressing. In a small bowl, whisk together the balsamic vinegar, honey, dijon mustard, minced garlic, and 2 tablespoons of olive oil. Set aside.
In a large bowl, combine the chopped kale and the roasted sweet potato wedges.
Add the dressing to the bowl and mix well to combine.
Divide the salad onto 4 plates, sprinkle with pomegranate seeds, and serve.

Nutrition Facts per serving
200 calories | 11g fat | 26g carbohydrates | 3g protein

Cauliflower and Carrot Salad with Raisins and Walnuts

Preparation Time: 20 minutes | Cooking Time: 25 minutes | Serving Size: 4

Ingredients:
1 head of cauliflower, chopped into bite-sized pieces
4 carrots, peeled and chopped into bite-sized pieces
2 tablespoons olive oil
Salt and pepper, to taste
1/2 cup raisins
1/2 cup chopped walnuts
2 tablespoons lemon juice
2 tablespoons honey
2 tablespoons Dijon mustard
1/4 cup chopped fresh parsley

Instructions:
Preheat oven to 400°F (200°C).
In a large bowl, combine the cauliflower, carrots, olive oil, salt, and pepper.
Spread the mixture evenly on a baking sheet and roast for 25 minutes, or until the vegetables are tender and slightly browned.
In another bowl, whisk together the lemon juice, honey, and Dijon mustard.
Add the roasted vegetables to the bowl with the dressing and stir to combine.
Stir in the raisins, walnuts, and parsley.
Serve the salad warm or at room temperature.

Nutrition Facts (per serving):
Calories: 259 | Total Fat: 16 g | Saturated Fat: 2 g | Trans Fat: 0 g | Cholesterol: 0 mg | Sodium: 128 mg | Total Carbohydrates: 30 g | Dietary Fiber: 5 g | Sugars: 20 g | Protein: 5 g | Vitamin D: 0 % | Calcium: 7 % | Iron: 8 %

Broccoli and Cheddar Salad with Bacon and Sunflower Seeds

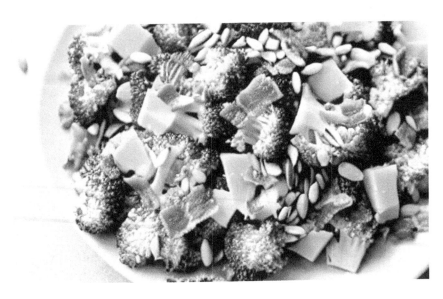

Preparation Time | Cooking Time | Serving Size: 15-20 minutes | 15-20 minutes | 4-6 servings

Ingredients:
4 cups broccoli florets
1 cup shredded cheddar cheese
8 strips bacon, cooked and chopped
1/2 cup sunflower seeds
1/2 cup mayonnaise
2 tablespoons apple cider vinegar
2 tablespoons honey
1/4 teaspoon salt
1/4 teaspoon black pepper

Instructions:
Preheat oven to 375°F (190°C).
Cook broccoli florets in boiling water for 4-5 minutes until tender, then drain and rinse with cold water to stop the cooking process.
In a large bowl, mix together the cooked broccoli, cheddar cheese, bacon, and sunflower seeds.
In a separate bowl, whisk together the mayonnaise, apple cider vinegar, honey, salt, and pepper.
Pour the dressing over the broccoli mixture and toss to combine.
Bake for 15-20 minutes, until cheese is melted and bubbly.
Serve and enjoy!

Nutrition Facts (per serving, based on 6 servings):
Calories: 400 | Fat: 34g | Saturated Fat: 8g | Cholesterol: 38mg | Sodium: 597mg | Carbohydrates: 14g | Fiber: 3g | Sugar: 9g | Protein: 13g

Chickpea and Feta Salad with Red Bell Pepper and Cucumber

Preparation time: 10 minutes | Cooking time: 0 minutes | Serving size: 4

Ingredients:
1 can chickpeas, drained and rinsed
1 red bell pepper, diced
1 cucumber, peeled and diced
1/2 cup crumbled feta cheese
2 tablespoons chopped fresh parsley
2 tablespoons lemon juice
2 tablespoons olive oil
Salt and pepper, to taste

Instructions:
In a large bowl, combine the chickpeas, red bell pepper, cucumber, feta cheese, and parsley.
In a small bowl, whisk together the lemon juice, olive oil, salt, and pepper.
Pour the dressing over the chickpea mixture and toss to combine.
Serve chilled or at room temperature.

Nutrition facts (per serving):
Calories: 285 | Total Fat: 19g | Saturated Fat: 7g | Cholesterol: 28mg | Sodium: 523mg | Total Carbohydrates: 19g | Dietary Fiber: 5g | Sugar: 4g | Protein: 10g

Cucumber and Tomato Salad with Feta Cheese and Herbs

Preparation Time: 15 minutes | Cooking Time: 0 minutes | Serving Size: 4

Ingredients:
2 large cucumbers, sliced
2 large tomatoes, chopped
4 oz feta cheese, crumbled
2 tablespoons chopped fresh parsley
2 tablespoons chopped fresh basil
1 tablespoon olive oil
1 tablespoon red wine vinegar
Salt and pepper to taste

Instructions:
In a large bowl, combine sliced cucumbers and chopped tomatoes.
Sprinkle crumbled feta cheese over the vegetables.

Add chopped parsley and basil to the bowl.

In a small bowl, whisk together olive oil and red wine vinegar. Season with salt and pepper to taste.

Pour the dressing over the salad and gently toss everything together.

Serve the salad immediately, or cover and refrigerate until ready to serve.

Nutrition Facts per Serving:

Calories: 162 | Fat: 12 g | Carbohydrates: 9 g | Protein: 7 g | Fiber: 2 g | Sodium: 474 mg

Asparagus and Avocado Salad with Hard-Boiled Eggs

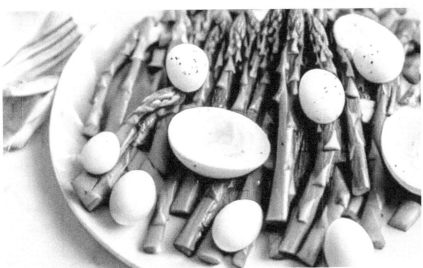

Preparation Time: 15 minutes | Cooking Time: 10 minutes | Serving Size: 4

Ingredients:

1 lb asparagus, trimmed

2 ripe avocados, diced

4 large eggs, hard-boiled and chopped

2 tbsp extra virgin olive oil

1 lemon, juiced

Salt and pepper to taste

Fresh herbs such as basil, parsley, or cilantro (optional)

Instructions:

Preheat oven to 400°F. Line a baking sheet with parchment paper.

Spread the asparagus on the prepared baking sheet and drizzle with 1 tbsp of the olive oil. Season with salt and pepper.

Roast for 10 minutes or until the asparagus is tender. Remove from oven and let it cool.

In a large bowl, gently mix together the roasted asparagus, diced avocados, hard-boiled eggs, lemon juice, remaining olive oil, and any herbs of your choice. Season with salt and pepper to taste.

Serve immediately or chill in the refrigerator until ready to serve.

Nutrition Facts (per serving):
Calories: 300 | Fat: 25g | Saturated Fat: 3.5g | Cholesterol: 186mg | Sodium: 123mg | Carbohydrates: 15g | Fiber: 8g | Sugar: 4g | Protein: 12g

Apple and Celery Salad with Walnuts and Blue Cheese

Preparation Time | Cooking Time | Serving Size: 15 minutes | 0 minutes | 4

Ingredients:
2 medium apples, cored and chopped
4 stalks of celery, sliced
1/2 cup walnuts, chopped
1/2 cup blue cheese, crumbled
2 tablespoons lemon juice
2 tablespoons olive oil
Salt and pepper, to taste

Instructions:
In a large bowl, combine the chopped apples, sliced celery, chopped walnuts, and crumbled blue cheese.
In a separate small bowl, whisk together the lemon juice, olive oil, salt, and pepper.
Pour the dressing over the salad ingredients and toss to combine.
Serve the salad immediately or chill in the refrigerator until ready to serve.

Nutrition Facts (per serving) |
Calories: 294 | Fat: 25 g | Saturated Fat: 7 g | Cholesterol: 24 mg | Sodium: 378 mg | Carbohydrates: 15 g | Fiber: 4 g | Sugar: 9 g | Protein: 8 g

Butternut Squash and Cranberry Salad with Feta Cheese

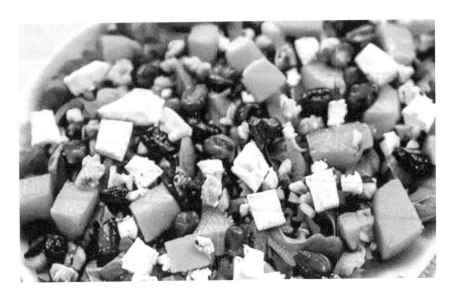

Preparation Time: 15 minutes | Cooking Time: 30 minutes | Serving Size: 4

Ingredients:
2 pounds butternut squash, peeled and cubed
1 cup fresh cranberries
2 tablespoons olive oil
Salt and pepper, to taste
4 ounces crumbled feta cheese
2 tablespoons chopped walnuts
1/4 cup balsamic vinaigrette

Instructions:
Preheat the oven to 400°F (200°C).

In a large bowl, mix the butternut squash and cranberries with the olive oil, salt, and pepper.

Transfer the mixture to a baking sheet and roast for 25-30 minutes, or until the squash is tender and lightly browned.

In a large serving bowl, mix the roasted butternut squash and cranberries with the feta cheese, walnuts, and balsamic vinaigrette.

Serve immediately or chill until ready to serve.

Nutrition Facts per Serving
Total Fat: 23g | Saturated Fat: 6g | Cholesterol: 22mg | Sodium: 393mg | Carbohydrates: 29g | Fiber: 5g | Sugar: 8g | Protein: 8g

Carrot and Ginger Salad with Peanuts and Cilantro

Preparation time: 10 minutes | Cooking time: 15 minutes | Serving size: 4

Ingredients:
4 large carrots, peeled and grated
1 inch piece of ginger, peeled and grated
1/4 cup peanuts, chopped
1/4 cup cilantro, chopped
2 tablespoons olive oil
2 tablespoons rice vinegar
1 tablespoon honey
1/2 teaspoon salt
Freshly ground black pepper to taste

Instructions:
Preheat oven to 400°F (200°C).

In a bowl, mix together grated carrots, ginger, peanuts, and cilantro.

In a small bowl, whisk together olive oil, rice vinegar, honey, salt, and pepper.

Toss the carrot mixture with the dressing until well coated.

Spread the mixture evenly on a baking sheet. Roast in the oven for 15 minutes or until the carrots are tender and lightly browned.

Serve the salad warm or at room temperature, garnished with additional cilantro and peanuts if desired.

Nutrition Facts per serving:
Calories: 204 | Total Fat: 16 g | Saturated Fat: 2 g | Cholesterol: 0 mg | Sodium: 382 mg | Total Carbohydrates: 16 g | Dietary Fiber: 3 g | Sugars: 10 g | Protein: 4 g

Roasted Vegetable Salad with Quinoa and Feta Cheese

Preparation Time: 30 minutes | Cooking Time: 45 minutes | Serving Size: 4-6

Ingredients:
2 medium sized eggplants, sliced
2 medium sized bell peppers, sliced
2 medium sized zucchinis, sliced
1 large red onion, sliced
1/4 cup olive oil
Salt and pepper, to taste
1 cup quinoa, cooked
4 ounces feta cheese, crumbled
2 tablespoons red wine vinegar
1/4 cup fresh parsley, chopped
1 lemon, juiced

Instructions:
Preheat oven to 400°F (200°C).
Line a baking sheet with parchment paper.
In a large bowl, mix together the eggplants, bell peppers, zucchinis, and onion.
Add in the olive oil, salt, and pepper and mix well.
Transfer the vegetables to the prepared baking sheet and bake for 25-30 minutes, until tender and slightly charred.
In a large bowl, mix together the cooked quinoa, feta cheese, red wine vinegar, parsley, lemon juice, and roasted vegetables.
Serve and enjoy!

Nutrition Facts per Serving (based on 6 servings)
Calories: 350 | Total Fat: 24g | Saturated Fat: 8g | Cholesterol: 33mg | Sodium: 380mg | Total Carbohydrates: 27g | Dietary Fiber: 7g | Sugars: 7g | Protein: 12g.

Grilled Zucchini and Tomato Salad with Feta Cheese and Basil

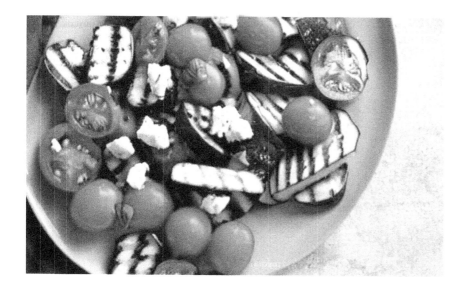

Preparation time: 10 minutes | Cooking time: 15 minutes | Serves: 4

Ingredients:
2 medium zucchini, sliced lengthwise
2 medium tomatoes, sliced
2 tablespoons olive oil
Salt and pepper, to taste
4 oz crumbled feta cheese
1/4 cup fresh basil leaves, chopped
For the vinaigrette:
2 tablespoons red wine vinegar
2 tablespoons olive oil
1 teaspoon honey
Salt and pepper, to taste

Instructions:
Preheat the grill to high heat.
Brush both sides of the zucchini and tomato slices with 2 tablespoons of olive oil, season with salt and pepper.
Place the zucchini and tomato slices on the grill and cook for about 7-8 minutes on each side, until charred and tender.
In a small bowl, whisk together the red wine vinegar, 2 tablespoons of olive oil, honey, salt, and pepper to make the vinaigrette.
In a large serving bowl, place the grilled zucchini and tomato slices. Sprinkle with crumbled feta cheese and chopped basil leaves.
Pour the vinaigrette over the salad and toss to combine. Serve immediately.
Nutrition facts (per serving):
Calories: 280 | Fat: 22g | Carbohydrates: 14g | Protein: 9g | Sodium: 430mg | Fiber: 3g | Sugar: 8g.

Broccoli and Raisin Salad with Almonds and Dried Cranberries

Preparation time: 20 minutes | Cooking time: 10 minutes | Serves: 4

Ingredients:
4 cups of broccoli florets, chopped
1/2 cup of raisins
1/2 cup of sliced almonds
1/2 cup of dried cranberries
1/2 cup of mayonnaise
2 tbsp of white wine vinegar
Salt and pepper to taste
Lettuce leaves (optional)

Instructions:
In a large bowl, combine the broccoli florets, raisins, almonds, and dried cranberries.
In a separate small bowl, whisk together the mayonnaise, white wine vinegar, salt and pepper.
Pour the dressing over the broccoli mixture and stir until evenly coated.
Cover the bowl and refrigerate the salad for at least 30 minutes to let the flavors meld.
Serve the salad on a bed of lettuce leaves, if desired.

Nutrition Facts (per serving):
Calories: 220 | Fat: 16g | Saturated Fat: 2g | Cholesterol: 5mg | Sodium: 330mg | Carbohydrates: 22g |
Fiber: 4g | Sugar: 15g | Protein: 4g

Cabbage and Carrot Slaw with Yogurt Dressing

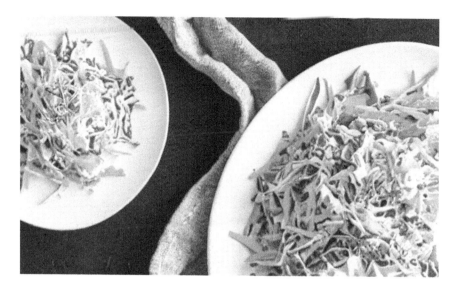

Preparation Time | Cooking Time | Serving Size: 20 minutes | 0 minutes | 6

Ingredients:
4 cups shredded green cabbage
2 cups grated carrots
1/4 cup plain Greek yogurt
2 tablespoons mayonnaise
2 tablespoons apple cider vinegar
1 tablespoon honey
Salt and pepper to taste
1/4 cup chopped fresh dill

Instructions:
In a large bowl, mix together the shredded cabbage and grated carrots.
In a separate bowl, whisk together the Greek yogurt, mayonnaise, apple cider vinegar, honey, salt, and pepper until well combined.
Pour the dressing over the cabbage mixture and toss to coat.
Add in the chopped dill and stir to combine.
Chill the slaw in the refrigerator for at least 30 minutes before serving.

Nutrition Facts (per serving):
Calories: 110 | Total Fat: 8g | Saturated Fat: 1.5g | Cholesterol: 5mg | Sodium: 170mg | Total Carbohydrates: 11g | Dietary Fiber: 3g | Sugar: 7g | Protein: 2g

Mixed Greens Salad with Grilled Chicken, Avocado and Grape Tomatoes

Preparation Time: 15 minutes | Cooking Time: 15 minutes | Serving Size: 4

Ingredients:
8 cups mixed greens
1 lb. boneless, skinless chicken breasts
1 avocado, diced
1 pint grape tomatoes, halved
1/4 cup olive oil
2 tbsp. balsamic vinegar
1 tsp. Dijon mustard
Salt and pepper to taste

Instructions:
Heat grill to medium-high heat.
Season the chicken breasts with salt and pepper, then grill for about 6 to 7 minutes per side, or until fully cooked. Remove from heat and let cool for 5 minutes before slicing into bite-sized pieces.
In a small bowl, whisk together the olive oil, balsamic vinegar, Dijon mustard, salt, and pepper to make the dressing.
In a large bowl, combine the mixed greens, grilled chicken, diced avocado, and halved grape tomatoes.
Pour the dressing over the salad and gently toss to combine.
Serve immediately, garnished with additional salt and pepper if desired.

Nutrition Facts per serving:
Calories: 463 | Fat: 35g | Carbohydrates: 17g | Protein: 26g | Sodium: 259mg | Fiber: 6g

Soup

Creamy Butternut Squash Soup

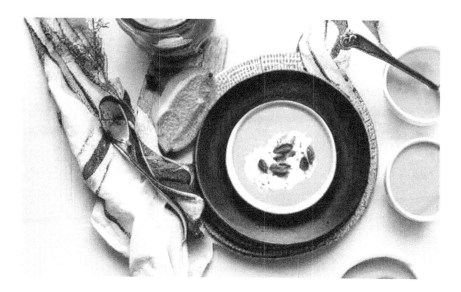

Preparation time: 10 minutes | Cooking time: 35 minutes | Serving size: 4-6

Ingredients:

1 large butternut squash (peeled, seeded and cubed)
1 onion, chopped
2 garlic cloves, minced
4 cups vegetable broth
1 tsp salt
1 tsp black pepper
1 tsp dried thyme
1 tsp dried rosemary
1/2 cup heavy cream
Fresh thyme or rosemary, for garnish (optional)

Instructions:

In a large pot, heat some oil over medium heat. Add the onion and garlic and cook until softened, about 5 minutes.

Add the butternut squash, vegetable broth, salt, pepper, dried thyme and rosemary to the pot.

Bring to a boil, reduce heat and let simmer until the squash is tender, about 25-30 minutes.

Remove from heat and let cool for a few minutes.

Use an immersion blender or transfer the soup to a blender and puree until smooth.

Return the soup to the pot and stir in the heavy cream.

Heat the soup over low heat until heated through.

Serve hot, garnished with fresh thyme or rosemary, if desired.

Nutrition facts (per serving, based on 4 servings):
Calories: 206 | Fat: 12g | Saturated Fat: 7g | Cholesterol: 39mg | Sodium: 1136mg | Carbohydrates: 22g | Fiber: 3g | Sugar: 4g | Protein: 3g

Gentle Chicken Noodle Soup

Preparation time: 20 minutes | Cooking time: 40 minutes | Serving size: 4-6

Ingredients:
1 large chicken breast (skinless and boneless)
8 cups of chicken broth
1 large onion, diced
2 cloves of garlic, minced
2 carrots, peeled and diced
2 celery stalks, diced
1 teaspoon dried thyme
2 cups of egg noodles
2 tablespoons of olive oil
Salt and pepper to taste
Fresh parsley for garnish

Instructions:
In a large pot, heat the olive oil over medium heat. Add the onion and garlic and cook until softened, about 3-4 minutes.
Add the chicken breast and cook until browned on both sides, about 3-4 minutes per side.
Add the chicken broth, carrots, celery, and thyme to the pot. Bring to a boil and reduce heat to low. Simmer until the chicken is cooked through, about 25 minutes.
Remove the chicken from the pot and let it cool. Shred the chicken into small pieces and set aside.
Add the egg noodles to the pot and cook until they are tender, about 10 minutes.
Add the shredded chicken back to the pot and season with salt and pepper to taste.
Serve the soup hot, garnished with fresh parsley if desired.

Nutrition facts per serving (based on 6 servings):
Calories: 234 | Total Fat: 9g | Saturated Fat: 2g | Cholesterol: 47mg | Sodium: 1432mg | Carbohydrates: 20g | Fiber: 2g | Sugar: 4g | Protein: 17g

Healthy Carrot Ginger Soup

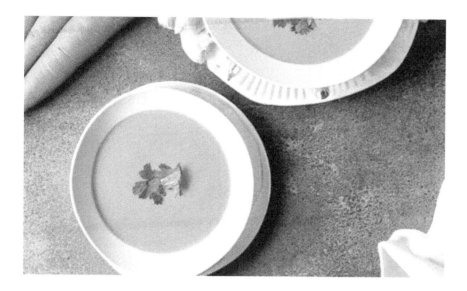

Preparation Time: 15 minutes | Cooking Time: 30 minutes | Serving Size: 4

Ingredients:

1 tablespoon of olive oil

1 medium onion, diced

3 garlic cloves, minced

2 inches of fresh ginger, peeled and grated

4 medium carrots, peeled and chopped

4 cups of chicken or vegetable broth

1 teaspoon of ground turmeric

1/2 teaspoon of salt

1/4 teaspoon of black pepper

1 cup of coconut milk

Instructions:

In a large pot, heat the olive oil over medium heat.

Add the onion and cook until softened, about 5 minutes.

Add the garlic and ginger and cook for an additional minute.

Add the chopped carrots, broth, turmeric, salt, and pepper to the pot.

Bring the mixture to a boil, then reduce the heat and let it simmer for 20-25 minutes, or until the carrots are soft.

Use an immersion blender or a regular blender to puree the soup until smooth.

Stir in the coconut milk and heat through.

Taste and adjust the seasoning as needed.

Serve the soup hot, garnished with fresh herbs or a drizzle of coconut milk, if desired.

Nutrition Facts (per serving):

Calories: 140 | Total Fat: 12g | Saturated Fat: 10g | Cholesterol: 0mg | Sodium: 540mg | Total Carbohydrates: 10g | Dietary Fiber: 3g | Sugar: 4g | Protein: 2g | Fat: 12g | Carbohydrates: 10g | Protein: 2g

Lighter Tomato Basil Soup

Preparation time | Cooking time | Serving size: 15 minutes | 30 minutes | 4

Ingredients:
2 tablespoons olive oil
1 onion, chopped
3 cloves of garlic, minced
4 medium-sized tomatoes, peeled and chopped
1 teaspoon dried basil
Salt and pepper to taste
1/2 cup heavy cream
4 cups chicken or vegetable broth
Fresh basil leaves for garnish

Instructions:
In a large pot, heat the olive oil over medium heat.
Add the chopped onion and cook until softened, about 5 minutes.
Add the minced garlic and cook for an additional minute.
Stir in the chopped tomatoes, dried basil, salt, and pepper. Cook for 10 minutes.
Add the broth and bring the mixture to a boil.
Reduce the heat and let it simmer for 15 minutes.
Carefully transfer the soup to a blender and puree until smooth.
Return the pureed soup back to the pot and stir in the heavy cream.
Heat the soup until warmed through, about 5 minutes.
Serve the soup hot, garnished with fresh basil leaves.

Nutrition Facts per serving:
Calories 210 | fat 18g | carbohydrates 11g | protein 4g | fiber 2g | sodium 270mg

Soothing Sweet Potato Soup

Preparation time: 10 minutes | Cooking time: 30 minutes | Serving size: 4

Ingredients:
2 tablespoons of olive oil
1 large onion, chopped
3 garlic cloves, minced
2 large sweet potatoes, peeled and diced
4 cups of chicken or vegetable broth
Salt and pepper to taste
1/4 teaspoon of ground nutmeg
1/4 teaspoon of smoked paprika
1 cup of half-and-half or heavy cream
2 tablespoons of chopped fresh parsley for garnish

Instructions:
In a large pot, heat the olive oil over medium heat. Add the onion and garlic and cook until softened, about 5 minutes.

Add the sweet potatoes, broth, salt, pepper, nutmeg, and paprika to the pot. Bring the mixture to a boil, then reduce heat and let it simmer for 20-25 minutes, or until the sweet potatoes are tender.

Use an immersion blender or transfer the mixture to a blender and puree until smooth. Return the puree to the pot.

Stir in the half-and-half or heavy cream and heat through.

Serve the soup hot, garnished with fresh parsley.

Nutrition Facts (per serving):
Calories: 250 | Total Fat: 19g | Saturated Fat: 7g | Cholesterol: 35mg | Sodium: 590mg | Total Carbohydrates: 19g | Dietary Fiber: 3g | Sugars: 7g | Protein: 3g | Vitamin A: 500% | Vitamin C: 4% | Calcium: 10% | Iron: 6%

Savory Lentil Soup

Preparation Time: 30 minutes | Cooking Time: 45 minutes | Serving Size: 4

Ingredients:
1 tablespoon olive oil
1 medium onion, chopped
3 cloves garlic, minced
1 teaspoon ground cumin
1 teaspoon ground coriander
1/2 teaspoon dried thyme
1/4 teaspoon red pepper flakes (optional)
3 cups vegetable broth
2 cups water
1 1/2 cups green lentils, rinsed and drained
2 large carrots, peeled and chopped
2 stalks celery, chopped
1 large potato, peeled and chopped
1 teaspoon salt
1/2 teaspoon black pepper
2 tablespoons fresh lemon juice

Instructions:
Heat the oil in a large saucepan over medium heat. Add the onion and garlic, and cook until softened, about 5 minutes.

Stir in the cumin, coriander, thyme, and red pepper flakes (if using). Cook for 1 minute, until fragrant.

Add the broth, water, lentils, carrots, celery, potato, salt, and black pepper. Bring to a boil, then reduce heat to low, cover, and simmer for 35 to 40 minutes, or until the lentils and vegetables are tender.

Stir in the lemon juice and taste for seasoning. Serve hot.

Nutrition Facts per serving
150 calories | 2g total fat | 0g saturated fat | 27g carbohydrates | 11g fiber | 9g protein

Refreshing Cucumber Soup

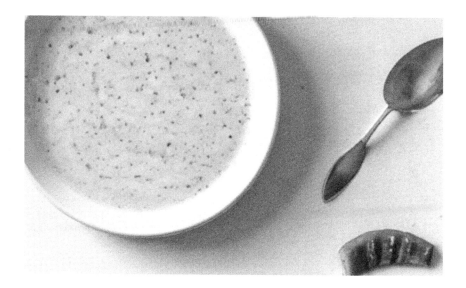

Preparation Time: 20 minutes | Cooking Time: 15 minutes | Serving Size: 4

Ingredients:

2 large cucumbers, peeled and chopped
1 medium onion, chopped
2 cloves of garlic, minced
2 cups of chicken or vegetable broth
1 cup of plain Greek yogurt
1/2 cup of fresh dill, chopped
1 tbsp of lemon juice
Salt and pepper, to taste
Croutons (optional)

Instructions:

In a large pot, heat a tablespoon of oil over medium heat. Add the onion and garlic and cook until softened, about 3-5 minutes.

Add the chopped cucumbers and cook for another 5 minutes.

Pour in the broth and bring the mixture to a boil. Reduce the heat and let it simmer for 10 minutes.

Use an immersion blender or a regular blender to puree the soup until smooth.

Stir in the yogurt, dill, lemon juice, salt, and pepper.

Taste the soup and adjust the seasoning as needed.

Serve the soup chilled, topped with croutons if desired.

Nutrition Facts (per serving, without croutons):

Calories: 95 | Fat: 4g | Carbohydrates: 10g | Protein: 6g | Sodium: 745mg | Fiber: 1g.

Rich Vegetable Broth

Preparation time: 20 minutes | Cooking time: 1 hour | Serving size: 8

Ingredients:
1 large onion, chopped
2 carrots, chopped
2 celery stalks, chopped
2 cloves garlic, minced
2 medium potatoes, chopped
1 cup chopped mushrooms
2 cups chopped kale or spinach
2 quarts (8 cups) water
2 tbsp olive oil
2 tsp salt
1 tsp black pepper
2 tbsp chopped fresh parsley (optional)

Instructions:
Heat the olive oil in a large pot over medium heat.
Add the onion, carrots, celery, garlic, and potatoes and cook until the vegetables are softened, about 10 minutes.
Stir in the mushrooms and kale and cook for another 5 minutes.
Add the water, salt, and pepper and bring to a boil.
Reduce heat and let the soup simmer for 45 minutes to an hour, until the vegetables are very tender.
Remove the soup from heat and let it cool for a few minutes.
Blend the soup with an immersion blender or transfer it to a blender and blend until smooth.
Return the soup to the pot and heat it over low heat until it is hot.
Serve with fresh parsley, if desired.

Nutrition Facts (per serving, based on 8 servings):
Calories: 116 | Total Fat: 5g | Saturated Fat: 1g | Cholesterol: 0mg | Sodium: 1057mg | Total Carbohydrates: 16g | Dietary Fiber: 3g | Sugar: 2g | Protein: 3g

Mild Leek and Potato Soup

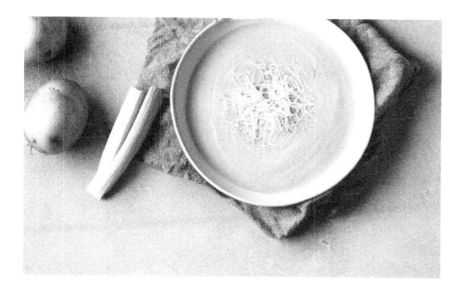

Preparation Time: 30 minutes | Cooking Time: 40 minutes | Serving Size: 4

Ingredients:
2 medium leeks, white and light green parts only, thinly sliced
2 medium potatoes, peeled and diced
4 cups vegetable broth
1 cup water
1 teaspoon salt
1/2 teaspoon black pepper
1/2 cup heavy cream (optional)
2 tablespoons butter
Fresh parsley or chives for garnish (optional)

Instructions:
In a large pot, melt the butter over medium heat.
Add the sliced leeks and cook until softened, about 5 minutes.
Add the diced potatoes, vegetable broth, water, salt, and pepper.
Bring the soup to a boil, then reduce the heat to low and let it simmer until the potatoes are tender, about 30 minutes.
Using an immersion blender or a regular blender, puree the soup until smooth.
If using heavy cream, stir it in now.
Taste and adjust seasoning as needed.
Serve hot, garnished with fresh parsley or chives if desired.

Nutrition Facts per serving (without cream):
Calories: 100 | Total Fat: 4g | Saturated Fat: 2g | Cholesterol: 10mg | Sodium: 1000mg | Total Carbohydrates: 16g | Dietary Fiber: 2g | Sugar: 2g | Protein: 2g

Tasty Zucchini Soup

Preparation time | Cooking time | Serving size: 15 minutes | 30 minutes | 4

Ingredients:
2 tablespoons of olive oil
2 medium zucchini, chopped
1 onion, chopped
3 cloves of garlic, minced
4 cups of vegetable broth
Salt and pepper, to taste
Fresh parsley, chopped (optional)

Instructions:
In a large pot, heat the olive oil over medium heat.
Add the chopped zucchini, onion, and garlic to the pot. Cook until softened, about 5 minutes.
Pour in the vegetable broth, and bring to a boil.
Reduce heat to low and let the soup simmer for about 20 minutes.
Using an immersion blender or a blender in batches, puree the soup until smooth.
Season with salt and pepper, to taste.
Serve the soup hot, garnished with fresh parsley if desired.

Nutrition facts (per serving)
Total Fat: 9g | Saturated Fat: 1g | Cholesterol: 0mg | Sodium: 640mg | Total Carbohydrates: 13g | Dietary Fiber: 2g | Sugar: 6g | Protein: 2g | Vitamin A: 4% | Vitamin C: 21% | Calcium: 4% | Iron: 6%

Nutritious Split Pea Soup

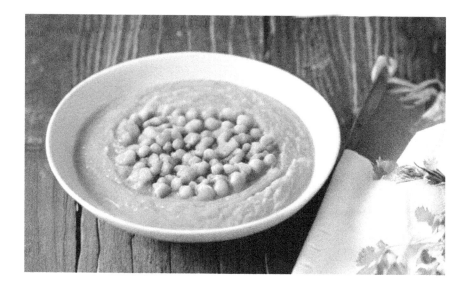

Preparation time: 20 minutes | Cooking time: 60 minutes | Serving size: 4

Ingredients:

1 pound dried green split peas
1 medium yellow onion, diced
2 carrots, peeled and diced
2 celery stalks, diced
3 cloves garlic, minced
4 cups chicken or vegetable broth
4 cups water
1 teaspoon dried thyme
1 teaspoon dried rosemary
1 bay leaf
Salt and pepper, to taste
Optional: diced ham or bacon for added flavor

Instructions:

Rinse the split peas and remove any small stones or debris.

In a large pot, heat a bit of oil over medium heat. Add the diced onion, carrots, celery and garlic and cook until the vegetables are tender and fragrant, about 5-7 minutes.

Add the broth, water, thyme, rosemary, bay leaf, split peas, and optional ham or bacon to the pot. Stir to combine.

Bring the mixture to a boil, then reduce the heat and let it simmer for 45-60 minutes, or until the split peas are soft and have fallen apart.

Remove the bay leaf and season with salt and pepper to taste.

Use an immersion blender or transfer the soup to a blender to puree until smooth. If the soup is too thick, add a bit more broth or water until it reaches your desired consistency.

Serve hot and enjoy!

Nutrition Facts per serving (4 servings):
Calories: 242 | Total Fat: 1g | Saturated Fat: 0g | Cholesterol: 0mg | Sodium: 551mg | Total Carbohydrates: 45g | Dietary Fiber: 16g | Sugar: 6g | Protein: 16g

Bright Broccoli and Cheese Soup

Preparation Time: 20 minutes | Cooking Time: 20 minutes | Serving Size: 4-6

Ingredients:
1 large head of broccoli, chopped
1 yellow onion, diced
3 cloves of garlic, minced
4 cups of chicken or vegetable broth
1 cup of heavy cream
1 cup of grated cheddar cheese
Salt and pepper, to taste
2 tbsp of butter or oil

Instructions:
Heat a large pot over medium heat and add the butter or oil.
Add the onion and garlic and cook until softened, about 5 minutes.
Add the broccoli to the pot and cook for another 5 minutes.
Pour in the broth and bring to a boil. Reduce heat to low and let simmer for 10 minutes.
Remove the pot from heat and let it cool for 5 minutes.
Blend the soup with an immersion blender or transfer to a blender and blend until smooth.
Return the soup to the pot and add the heavy cream. Heat the soup over low heat.
Gradually add the grated cheese and stir until melted.
Season the soup with salt and pepper, to taste.
Serve hot with crusty bread or croutons.

Nutrition Facts (per serving) | 1 serving (based on 6 servings) :
Calories: 359 | Fat: 28.5 g | Saturated Fat: 18.5 g | Cholesterol: 93 mg | Sodium: 648 mg | Carbohydrates: 13.2 g | Protein: 12.2 g

Wholesome Minestrone Soup

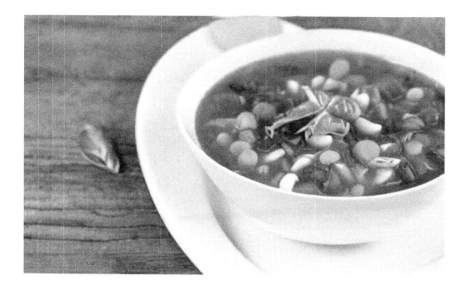

Preparation time: 20 minutes | Cooking time: 30 minutes | Serves: 4

Ingredients:
1 tbsp olive oil
1 large onion, chopped
2 garlic cloves, minced
2 carrots, peeled and diced
2 celery stalks, diced
2 large potatoes, peeled and diced
2 cups chopped tomatoes
4 cups chicken or vegetable broth
1 can (15 oz) of kidney beans, drained and rinsed
1 can (15 oz) of cannellini beans, drained and rinsed
1 cup uncooked elbow macaroni
2 cups chopped kale or spinach
2 tbsp fresh basil, chopped
Salt and pepper, to taste

Instructions:
In a large pot, heat the oil over medium heat. Add the onion and garlic and cook until soft and translucent, about 5 minutes.

Add the carrots, celery, and potatoes and cook until they start to soften, about 5-7 minutes.

Stir in the chopped tomatoes, broth, kidney beans, cannellini beans, and macaroni.

Bring the mixture to a boil, then reduce heat and let it simmer until the macaroni is cooked, about 10 minutes.

Stir in the kale or spinach and basil and cook until wilted, about 2-3 minutes.

Season with salt and pepper, to taste.

Serve hot and enjoy!

Nutrition Facts (per serving):
Calories: 324 | Fat: 5g | Saturated Fat: 1g | Cholesterol: 0mg | Sodium: 864mg | Carbohydrates: 57g | Fiber: 13g | Sugar: 7g | Protein: 16g

Hearty Bean and Vegetable Soup

Preparation Time: 20 minutes | Cooking Time: 40 minutes | Serving Size: 4

Ingredients:
1 tablespoon olive oil
1 medium onion, diced
2 garlic cloves, minced
2 medium carrots, diced
2 celery stalks, diced
1 large potato, diced
1 can of diced tomatoes (14.5 ounces)
4 cups of vegetable broth
1 can of kidney beans (15 ounces), drained and rinsed
1 can of corn (15 ounces), drained
1 teaspoon dried thyme
Salt and pepper, to taste

Instructions:
In a large pot, heat the olive oil over medium heat.
Add the onion and garlic, and cook until the onion is translucent, about 5 minutes.
Add the carrots, celery, and potato, and cook for 5 more minutes.
Add the diced tomatoes, vegetable broth, kidney beans, corn, and thyme, and bring to a boil.
Reduce the heat to low and let the soup simmer for 30 minutes, or until the vegetables are tender.
Season with salt and pepper to taste.
Serve hot and enjoy.

Nutrition Facts per serving:
Calories: 220 | Fat: 4g | Sodium: 470mg | Carbohydrates: 39g | Fiber: 9g | Protein: 11g

Rustic Cauliflower Soup

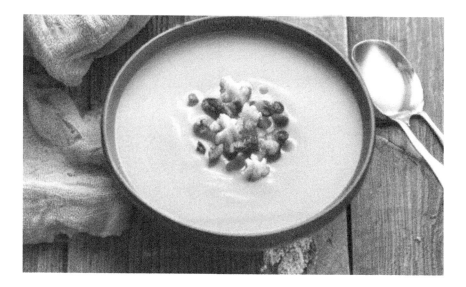

Preparation Time | Cooking Time | Serving Size: 15 minutes | 30 minutes | 6

Ingredients:

1 head of cauliflower, chopped
1 large onion, chopped
3 cloves of garlic, minced
4 cups of vegetable broth
2 cups of water
1 teaspoon of dried thyme
1 teaspoon of dried basil
Salt and pepper, to taste
2 tablespoons of olive oil
Fresh parsley for garnish (optional)

Instructions:

Heat the olive oil in a large pot over medium heat.
Add the onion and garlic, and cook until the onion is translucent and fragrant, about 5 minutes.
Add the cauliflower, vegetable broth, water, thyme, basil, salt and pepper to the pot. Stir to combine.
Bring the soup to a boil, then reduce heat to low and cover the pot.
Simmer the soup for 25-30 minutes, or until the cauliflower is tender.
Use an immersion blender to puree the soup until smooth, or transfer the soup to a blender and puree in batches.
Return the pureed soup to the pot, and heat through if necessary.
Serve the soup hot, garnished with fresh parsley if desired.

Nutrition Facts (per serving, based on 6 servings)

Calories: 114 | Fat: 7.2g | Saturated Fat: 1.1g | Cholesterol: 0mg | Sodium: 480mg | Carbohydrates: 12.4g | Fiber: 4.7g | Sugar: 4.4g | Protein: 4.2g

Vibrant Pea and Mint Soup

Preparation time: 15 minutes | Cooking time: 25 minutes | Serving size: 4

Ingredients:
1 tbsp olive oil
1 onion, chopped
2 cloves garlic, minced
2 medium carrots, chopped
2 potatoes, chopped
4 cups fresh or frozen peas
4 cups vegetable broth
1/2 cup fresh mint leaves
Salt and pepper to taste
Greek yogurt or sour cream, for serving (optional)

Instructions:
Heat the olive oil in a large saucepan over medium heat.

Add the onion and garlic and cook until the onion is soft and translucent, about 5 minutes.

Add the carrots, potatoes, peas, and vegetable broth to the saucepan and bring to a boil.

Reduce heat to low and let simmer for 20 minutes or until the vegetables are tender.

Add the mint leaves and let the soup continue to simmer for an additional 5 minutes.

Use an immersion blender or transfer the soup to a blender and puree until smooth.

Season with salt and pepper to taste.

Serve with a dollop of Greek yogurt or sour cream, if desired.

Nutrition Facts per serving (based on 4 servings):
Calories: 189 | Fat: 7g | Saturated Fat: 1g | Cholesterol: 0mg | Sodium: 735mg | Carbohydrates: 28g | Fiber: 8g | Sugar: 8g | Protein: 8g

Warm Chickpea and Spinach Soup

Preparation Time: 15 minutes | Cooking Time: 30 minutes | Serving Size: 4

Ingredients:
1 tablespoon olive oil
1 medium onion, chopped
2 cloves garlic, minced
1 teaspoon ground cumin
1/2 teaspoon smoked paprika
1/4 teaspoon red pepper flakes
4 cups vegetable broth
1 can chickpeas, drained and rinsed
1 cup chopped fresh spinach
Salt and black pepper, to taste
Fresh lemon juice, for serving (optional)

Instructions:
In a large saucepan, heat the olive oil over medium heat.
Add the onion and garlic and cook until softened, about 5 minutes.
Stir in the cumin, paprika, and red pepper flakes and cook for 1 minute.
Pour in the vegetable broth, chickpeas, and spinach and bring to a simmer.
Reduce heat to low and let the soup cook for 15 minutes.
Season with salt and black pepper to taste.
Serve the soup with a squeeze of lemon juice, if desired.

Nutrition Facts per serving (based on 4 servings):
Calories 164 | Fat: 6g | Sodium: 748 mg | Carbohydrates: 25g | Fiber: 8g | Protein: 8g

Nourishing Kale and Quinoa Soup

Preparation Time: 15 minutes | Cooking Time: 30 minutes | Serving Size: 4-6

Ingredients:
1 tbsp olive oil
1 large onion, chopped
2 cloves garlic, minced
2 large carrots, chopped
2 celery stalks, chopped
2 tsp ground cumin
1 tsp dried thyme
1 tsp dried basil
4 cups vegetable broth
1 cup water
1 cup quinoa, rinsed
4 cups chopped kale
Salt and pepper to taste

Instructions:
Heat the olive oil in a large pot over medium heat.
Add the onion and garlic, and cook until softened, about 5 minutes.
Add the carrots and celery and cook for another 5 minutes.
Stir in the cumin, thyme, and basil, and cook for 1 minute.
Pour in the broth, water, and quinoa, and bring to a boil.
Reduce heat to low, cover and simmer for 20 minutes, or until the quinoa is cooked.
Stir in the kale and cook until wilted, about 5 minutes.
Season with salt and pepper to taste.
Serve hot.

Nutrition Facts (per serving):
Calories: 186 | Fat: 6g | Saturated Fat: 1g | Cholesterol: 0mg | Sodium: 1001mg | Carbohydrates: 29g | Fiber: 5g | Sugar: 3g | Protein: 7g

Flavorful Spinach and Rice Soup

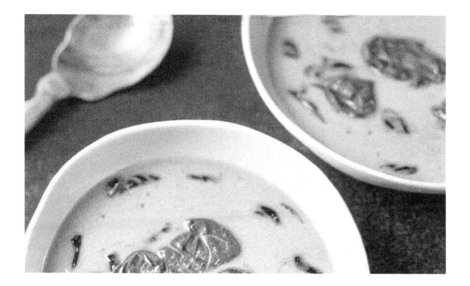

Preparation Time: 10 minutes | Cooking Time: 30 minutes | Servings: 4

Ingredients:
1 tablespoon olive oil
1 onion, chopped
2 cloves garlic, minced
4 cups chicken or vegetable broth
1 cup long-grain white rice
6 cups baby spinach
Salt and pepper, to taste
2 tablespoons lemon juice
Fresh parsley, chopped (optional)

Instructions:
Heat the oil in a large saucepan over medium heat.
Add the onion and cook until soft, about 5 minutes.
Add the garlic and cook for another minute.
Add the broth, rice, and a pinch of salt and pepper. Bring to a boil.
Reduce the heat and let simmer for 20 minutes, or until the rice is cooked.
Add the spinach and let cook until wilted, about 2-3 minutes.
Stir in the lemon juice.
Serve hot, garnished with fresh parsley if desired.

Nutrition Facts (per serving):
Calories: 220 | Total Fat: 5g | Saturated Fat: 1g | Cholesterol: 0mg | Sodium: 800mg | Total Carbohydrates: 40g | Dietary Fiber: 2g | Sugars: 2g | Protein: 7g

Filling Butternut Squash and Apple Soup

Preparation Time: 30 minutes | Cooking Time: 45 minutes | Serving Size: 4-6

Ingredients:
1 large butternut squash, peeled and diced
2 medium apples, peeled and diced
1 onion, chopped
2 garlic cloves, minced
4 cups chicken or vegetable broth
1 tsp dried thyme
1 tsp dried sage
Salt and pepper to taste
Optional: 1/2 cup heavy cream, for a creamy version

Instructions:
In a large pot, heat 1 tbsp of olive oil over medium heat. Add the chopped onion and cook until it starts to soften, around 5 minutes.
Add the minced garlic and cook for another minute.
Add the diced butternut squash and apples to the pot, along with the dried thyme, sage, and salt and pepper. Cook for 5 minutes, stirring occasionally.
Pour in the broth and bring to a boil. Reduce the heat to low and let the soup simmer for 30-35 minutes, or until the squash and apples are very soft.
Using an immersion blender or transfer the soup in batches to a blender or food processor, puree the soup until it is smooth.
If desired, stir in the heavy cream.
Serve the soup hot with crusty bread or crackers.

Nutrition Facts per serving (without heavy cream):
Calories: 160 kcal | Total Fat: 1 g | Saturated Fat: 0 g | Cholesterol: 0 mg | Sodium: 580 mg | Total Carbohydrates: 39 g | Dietary Fiber: 7 g | Sugars: 12 g | Protein: 4 g

Conclusion

In this book, we have explored a variety of delicious and nutritious recipes that are suitable for those without a gallbladder. We have highlighted the importance of consuming low-fat, high-fiber foods, as well as incorporating plenty of fruits and vegetables into the diet. Through these recipes, we hope that individuals with this condition can find relief from symptoms and continue to lead a healthy, fulfilling life.

As a reminder, it is important to always consult with a healthcare provider before making any major changes to your diet. Additionally, it is essential to monitor your body's reaction to the foods you consume and adjust accordingly.

In conclusion, the No Gallbladder Diet Cookbook provides a resource for individuals to enjoy a variety of flavors and ingredients, all while maintaining a healthy and balanced diet. We hope that this cookbook will serve as a helpful guide for those without a gallbladder, and encourage them to experiment and discover new, delicious dishes.

DOWNLOAD HERE
THE 2 EBOOK BONUS
And
COLOR VERSION OF THE BOOK

Or copy and paste this url:

https://bit.ly/2bonusnogallbladderwilliamdean

Made in the USA
Coppell, TX
17 May 2023

16976718R00063